# ATHLETIC
# ABs

Scott Cole
Tom Seabourne

**Human Kinetics**

**Library of Congress Cataloging-in-Publication Data**

Cole, Scott, 1962-
  Athletic abs / Scott Cole, Tom Seabourne.
  p. cm.
  ISBN 0-7360-4121-4 (pbk.)
  1. Abdominal exercises.  2. Physical fitness.  I. Seabourne, Thomas.
II. Title.
  GV508 .C66  2003
  613.7'1--dc21

2002004146

ISBN: 0-7360-4121-4

Acquisitions Editor: Martin Barnard
Developmental Editor: Cynthia McEntire
Assistant Editor: John Wentworth
Copyeditor: Karen Bojda
Proofreader: Jennifer L. Davis
Graphic Designer: Robert Reuther
Graphic Artist: Francine Hamerski
Photo Manager: Tom Roberts
Cover Designer: Jack W. Davis
Cover photo of Scott Cole: Scott Ashton
Photographer (interior): Tom Roberts
Models: Bylle Fortier, Heather Nelson, Adam Gockel, and Daniel Head
Art Manager: Carl D. Johnson
Illustrator: Argosy Publishing
Printer: Versa Press

Printed in the United States of America   10 9 8 7 6 5 4 3 2 1

**Human Kinetics**
Web site: www.HumanKinetics.com

*United States:* Human Kinetics
P.O. Box 5076
Champaign, IL 61825-5076
800-747-4457
e-mail: humank@hkusa.com

*Canada:* Human Kinetics
475 Devonshire Road Unit 100
Windsor, ON N8Y 2L5
800-465-7301 (in Canada only)
e-mail: orders@hkcanada.com

*Europe:* Human Kinetics
107 Bradford Road
Stanningley
Leeds LS28 6AT, United Kingdom
+44 (0) 113 255 5665
e-mail: hk@hkeurope.com

*Australia:* Human Kinetics
57A Price Avenue
Lower Mitcham, South Australia 5062
08 8277 1555
e-mail: liahka@senet.com.au

*New Zealand:* Human Kinetics
P.O. Box 105-231, Auckland Central
09-523-3462
e-mail: hkp@ihug.co.nz

# ATHLETIC
# ABs

# contents

# preface

The working title for this book originally was *The Last Word on Abs*. What a great title, we thought, until we both realized that we were buying into that incredibly seductive male know-it-all expert thing that we both inherently despise and have worked so hard to overcome. You know—that beating-the-chest "Popeye syndrome" of drinking your milk (which now gives us gas), eating your spinach (which we recommend even though it gives you gas), keeping your real emotions inside, and telling everybody else what to do.

In our defense, and in light of our ever-evolving 21st-century male egos, we humbly admit how incredibly pompous it was for us to even think of claiming we had the last word on abs, as if we were bored, unchallenged, and unimpressed with everything else that had been written on abs, washboard abs, and tummies thus far. In reality, deep below our chiseled, manly facades, we knew indeed that this would most likely not be the last word on abs and surely would not be our last word on abs either. So acknowledging our own fallibility but still intrigued by the sequel possibility of *The Total, Absolute Last Word on Abs* and the follow-up *OK, We Lied, There Is More on Abs*, we forged ahead reluctantly in search of a new title.

Then came the vision: *Athletic Abs*. Picture this Hollywood promo: "In a world full of abdominal imposters, armed only with core strength and their six-packs, two men stand alone . . . Scott Cole and Tom Seabourne." Tom Cruise, Brad Pitt, and Christian Bale are already fighting for the two slots to portray us as two ego-less guys on a mission to save the world. We wish all three of them the best of luck. There are no losers, though, in this lusty tale of great and powerful abs.

If you are smiling, that makes us happy, and if you are laughing out loud, you are truly on your way to the best abs on earth. Laughing is a great way to work your abs, and if the truth were known, we are actually a little bored. We are bored and professionally frustrated by watching people train ineffectively when we know some fundamental training secrets that can change the way people train not only their abs but their entire body and mind. Rather than complain about the abdominal duping of the consumer, we decided to bring you *Athletic Abs*.

If you have been looking for a solution to get rid of your gut, you have found it, although the solution is not primarily the book or the exercises themselves. It is the personal training experience you will find here, over 45 years of combined professional training experience between us.

This book gives you real tools to build new healthier ways of living through exercise, stress reduction, and overall mental and spiritual body awareness. (And you thought we were just going to give you a couple of ab workouts and send you home.) You can take it at six-pack surface value and see results, but if you want to move up a notch on the awareness scale to truly experience what core strength is all about, read on to see how we have trained and maintained our physiques with no drugs, crazy supplements, useless ab products, or surgery.

Sports have always been a great way for people to express themselves. They are safe (usually) and fun (hopefully); scientific research demonstrates the need for bodily activity. Tom, a complete sportsman, martial artist, and athlete, shares this experience: "When I was 11 years old, I was tall and skinny. All of my karate buddies marveled at my abdominal development. They thought I trained my abs hours per week. Little did they know, I never conventionally trained my abs. Punching and kicking developed my abs more than any sit-up or crunch routine."

It is important to understand the function of our core. Scott has a similar story in college at the University of Texas as head cheerleader: "In order to make the squad at UT, all of the guys had to throw five standing back flips, diving onto the field between each flip to spell out T-E-X-A-S with our bodies. The full extension of my body, with the natural knee tuck to my chest and stabilizing force of my abs in a 'back tuck,' gave me some chiseled abs. They got really chiseled because I was not a natural gymnast so I had to crash a few times and train even harder."

We are not recommending that you eliminate crunches, get kicked in the gut, or crash trying to do back flips. We are (thank goodness) recommending some new, efficient, and more enjoyable ways to train.

When thinking about what is missing in most people's core/abdominal training, we look to the best abs on earth, literally: What do you think gymnasts, martial artists, divers, sprinters, cyclists, and surfers all have in common?

1. They all do 500 crunches daily.
2. They participate in secret abdominal conventions.
3. They all watched the same infomercial.
4. They all use core strength in their sports of choice.

If you chose answer 4, you are on your way to the best abs on earth. Whether your sport of choice is triathlons or carrying the groceries, there is something here for you. We want you to have fun, get in great shape, and inspire others to do the same.

# acknowledgments

*Athletic Abs* would not have been possible without my family, friends, students, and my very talented co-author, Tom Seabourne. Many thanks as well for the collaborative process with Martin Barnard, Cynthia McEntire, and Tom Roberts at Human Kinetics, allowing us to take the study of the body and all of its intricacies to new heights. I joyfully thank Nature, God, and the Universe (which are all One to me) for the gift of life, creativity, and movement.

—SCOTT COLE

I want to thank my mother, brother, and sister for their inspiration as fitness club owners in Allentown, Pennsylvania. Also, my motivation to pursue this exciting endeavor came from my wife and five children, who happily tested most of our core exercises. And without Cynthia McEntire of Human Kinetics and Scott Cole, *Athletic Abs* would never have happened. Scott was the brains behind the video and a huge part of the book. Scott's innovative wit and talent have made *Athletic Abs* a wonderful success.

—TOM SEABOURNE

# introduction

Choose your weapons. Actually, you already have your weapons: Just choose to turn your "ab" into abs. We want you to enjoy the emergence of your strong core as you experience the best abs on earth.

Abdominal or core training used to be about crunches, twists, and sit-ups. The exercises in this book train your abs in a full-body workout, improving abdominal strength, muscular endurance, flexibility, body awareness, and mental toughness. The exercises in this book were inspired by sports training, innovative fitness practices, martial arts techniques, gymnastics, yoga, and tai chi.

*Athletic Abs* is the next generation of abdominal training. The exercises in this book take advantage of controlled instability. Although this sounds like a personal or psychological problem, controlled instability is merely our way to describe the safe core drills we present, drills that make your abs work harder to stabilize your body—that is, move from instability to stability—with less risk of injury.

In this program, you will learn to train your whole body as an integrated unit in addition to isolating core body parts. You may ask, "Are sit-ups and crunches bad?" They are not bad when done correctly. Doing only sit-ups and crunches, however, is a one-dimensional way to train and doesn't really address overall core conditioning, strength, flexibility, and functionality. Athletic strength and prowess will not improve through crunches alone. Sit-ups and crunches are performed on a flat floor. That means you develop your core strength at about 30 degrees of trunk flexion, and that is about it. Your hip flexors do the rest of the work to flex your spine, especially if you are one of those people who do crazed, momentum-flinging, thrill-seeking, tailbone-smashing, full sit-ups. Even if you are one of those, don't panic; you are in the right place for recovery. When you do your crunches, at least do them correctly (as shown in chapter 5); read the rest of the book for a more effective approach.

This book features a huge variety of standing, kneeling, seated, lengthening, knee-raising, midline-crossing, and stabilizing exercises, teaching you all about the abs, surrounding muscle groups, full-body core training, and more. Training only single components is missing the point of true core training. Our unique integrated drills will truly make your midsection a cut above, pun intended!

If your goal is for your abs to show (not an unreasonable goal), keep in mind that doing 10 million crunches will not make the layer of fat around your middle disappear. Cardiovascular fat-burning exercise (cardio interval-training drills) is required to reduce overall body fat. So even if your abs are undiscovered, seemingly requiring an archaeological expedition (like the discovery of Tut's tomb), fear not. You can train and become just as strong as someone who sports a six-pack. Actually, you have one, too; you just can't see it yet. By eating sensibly and increasing your activity to jump-start your metabolism, you'll feel, see, and unveil those long-lost abs sooner than you think! Follow the step-by-step exercises in *Athletic Abs* today and within a month you will notice a wonderful change in your body.

We also teach you correct body positioning and martial arts–inspired strength and resiliency techniques that both improve your posture and prevent lower-back pain. We provide a thorough series of stability exercises in which your arms and legs move in opposition around your center, emphasizing the importance of a strong, sturdy leg base and training your abs like never before.

Our series of yoga poses, gymnastic strength moves, and partner drills further demonstrate what this book is all about and are perhaps our finest illustration of real core strength. Some of the more advanced moves require guided preparation and, though they are safe to attempt, cannot be done effectively without real abdominal strength and flexibility. You will see and feel your improvement as you master these skills.

Full-range, short-range, mixed-range, and isometric core strengthening exercises are included in the program, along with an easy-to-understand explanation of the relationship between muscles. Understanding your anatomy is only part of the process. Common training questions are also answered along the way. Should you train your core first or last? Should you lift your legs or raise your torso first?

The American College of Sports Medicine (ACSM) recommends that programs such as this one be an integral part of an adult fitness program. This is because training does not just produce cosmetic benefits but delivers results you can feel as well as see. You can look forward to the following improvements in your health:

- Lower blood pressure
- Increased food transit time through the colon, which combats some types of cancer
- Increased bone density, which decreases your risk of osteoporosis
- Increased HDL cholesterol (the "good" kind)
- Decreased risk for diabetes. Additional muscle uses more oxygen and takes up extra sugar. Lower blood sugar levels are important for the prevention of type 2 diabetes.

Flexibility is often the forgotten component of fitness programs. We address stretching for comfort, muscle recovery, and balance. An inflexible body is most often an easily injured body, and we take you further on the flexibility scale than any other abs program.

In many of the exercises, we use an informal scale (levels 1, 2, and 3) to help you decide which exercises are appropriate for you based on your fitness level. The scale is based on the complexity and intensity of the exercise. Beginners should start with level 1 exercises; those who are more active and fit can progress to levels 2 and 3. Choose exercises that you feel comfortable with but that challenge your body. You shouldn't push yourself so hard that you hurt yourself, but you shouldn't go so easy you fall asleep either. At all times, use your best judgment in deciding how hard to train. Exercise compulsion and body obsession is not a healthy approach. Avoid pushing yourself to injury. Good training techniques are best implemented with a clear mind, a relaxed sense of body awareness, and disciplined dedication. Use common sense and caution when trying any new technique.

## HOW TO USE CORE TRAINING

You know you should follow a core-training program, but you don't know exactly when, how, or why to use it. You read all of the fitness magazines, but the information changes. How do you know what to do and when to do it?

Let us show you the way. Contained within these covers is a unique collection of exercises to improve your flexibility, tone your torso, strengthen your back, and increase your body awareness.

Make yourself a member of an elite group. Did you know that fewer than 20 percent of Americans work out regularly? The man or woman you just waved to on the bike was the same person you saw running yesterday. Few people create the time to train. Many people say they will try to work out later in the day but find other things to do instead. Your workout time is vital to your health and longevity.

How about getting jump-started first thing in the morning? Get up 30 minutes earlier, do your routine, and feel energized the rest of the day. Follow these 10 steps to peak performance:

1. Your alarm sounds; hit the five-minute snooze button.
2. Breathe fully as you mentally prepare for your workout.
3. Your alarm sounds again (no moaning!); open your eyes, ground your feet, and greet the morning with a good attitude.
4. Visit the restroom (make sure you are awake).
5. Drink a little water or fresh juice.
6. Put on the workout clothes that you set out the night before.
7. Warm up and begin your training program.
8. Relax with flexibility exercises.
9. Take a shower, feeling refreshed, energized, and pumped.
10. Eat a healthy breakfast and employ the posture tips throughout the day.

## REALISTIC GOALS

A mesomorphic body type (like Jean-Claude Van Damme) is one with well-defined muscles on the trunk and limbs. These people are broad in the shoulders and hips and narrow in the waist. They have a high muscle-to-fat ratio and often have ripped abs even without our program (but are they really happy?).

An endomorphic body type is rounder, softer, and more pear-shaped. These people generally know the true meaning of life, having had to deal with snotty-nosed insults from ignorant people. It is an untruth to assume that an endomorph cannot have a great looking, magnificently functioning body. These people have more fat surrounding their gluteals and thighs, their muscles are not well defined, and they possess a lower muscle-to-fat ratio, so they have to work a little harder to stay lean.

An ectomorphic body type would look like Bruce Lee without muscles. Ectomorphs' bodies are long and rectangular, flat chested, slender in the hips, with no defined waist (pretty much the supermodel category). Ectomorphs generally have less muscle and relatively low body weight. This body type has a difficult time retaining muscle and must take in enough calories to achieve muscle definition.

It is important to admire and enjoy your own uniqueness, rather than obsess about what you are not. Being different is a great thing, not a tragedy. No matter what body type you possess, you will harvest the rewards of *Athletic Abs:* a leaner, stronger, more flexible body. You'll see the improvement in your outward appearance, but more important, you'll also feel the difference inside.

# UNDERSTANDING YOUR AB-SOLUTE POTENTIAL

You will see a noticeable improvement in your physique by following the program. You do not need to agonize your way to a disappointing end result. We employ the spiritual perspective of staying in the moment and enjoying and learning from your own process. With this philosophy, there is no failure. Students of the martial arts learn that with emotional, mental, and spiritual support of self, the body responds miraculously. In this book, we use these elements to tone and strenghten the core.

Our program is a multilevel process that you can enjoy without cluttering your life with deprivation diets, mysterious physique-enhancing supplements, and panicked scale watching. With all of that negativity behind you, you will begin to feel and understand the benefits of healthy eating and exercise. Fear-based fitness has no place in our program.

Passionate athletes know the feeling of letting go of fear, reaching a "runner's high," or "getting lost" in their sport of choice. If you don't know that feeling (but you will!), it is similar to playing outside all day long, as you did as a child without a care in the world. For example, as you are jumping up toward the basket for a perfect layup, you are most likely not thinking, "OK, my quads begin the movement; my energy is now flowing up through my body, abs stabilizing, arms extending, as the ball leaves my fingers." In those moments, it is your training and your attitude that really pay off, and they indeed become second nature. You will feel no hesitation as you make that layup a functional, joyful work of art . . . and an easy two points!

Enjoy your journey!

# TRAINING

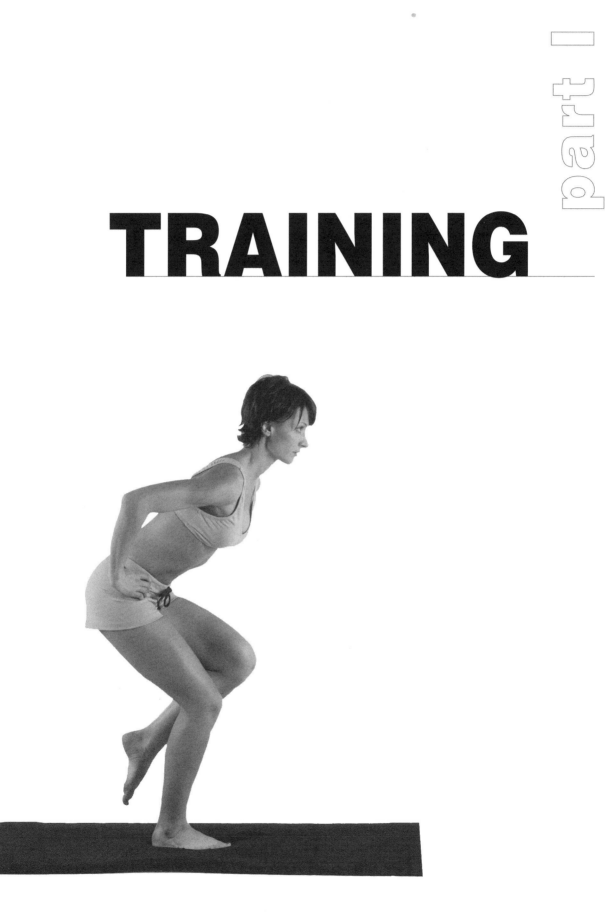

# part I

# BUILDING THE CORE:

## Find Your Center

Great athletes and martial artists tune in to their power center. The ancient Chinese martial art of tai chi teaches that internal force and awareness is centered below the navel, underneath the abs, in the "core" of the body. The core of an apple contains the seeds, just as the interior center of the body contains the life force. The word *core* is often defined as the innermost or most important part. This is also true of the human core. The midsection muscles are magnificently designed to surround, cover, and protect your innermost or most important part, your core.

Martial artists have known for centuries that true human power begins in the core. You can't break bricks and ward off opponents by having just strong arms and legs. Acclaimed martial artist Bruce Lee initiated his explosive punches and kicks from his mentally centered, well-trained core, allowing energy to flow through his strong and resilient body with unparalleled human force. He was a prime example of power and strength and, as a result of his high level of training, had incredible abs. We can't all be Bruce Lee, but we can learn a lot from martial arts training.

Visualization, innate body awareness, and mental preparation are part of martial arts training. Imagine that you are the highly skilled star of a blockbuster martial arts film (no special effects allowed). Visualize your abs lengthening, contracting, stabilizing with every movement and every breath. As you turn slowly, a crazed fan unexpectedly appears on the set, preparing to punch you in the abdomen. Because you maintain a relaxed, heightened state of martial awareness, you sense the blow coming and, rather than tensing your body and flexing your abdominal muscles (which would be a martial arts "no-no" of meeting force with force), you instead exhale quickly and forcefully, automatically contracting and protecting your abs as you turn your torso slightly to deflect the force. Think of a tree in the breeze, grounded but resilient. The solution requires an overall physical, mental, and spiritual awareness that naturally deflects danger away from your valuable core. The motivation of self-protection provides a powerful abdominal contraction.

Subtle but perceptible messages are often sent through core stability and strength. When you are centered and internally aware, your senses are heightened. For example, when you shake hands with someone, you can sense his or her strength and stability, an energy exchange between two people. A relaxed, strong handshake is more than just a squeeze of the hand; its strength comes from a strong core. Like a good hug or embrace, you feel energy, or "chi," when you shake hands. When you shake hands with someone familiar, it is possible to detect an altered mood without words at all; an intuitive message is sent. Even when you shake hands with someone you don't know, you make an intuitive and physical connection. Martial artists and intuitive, core-centered people live by this, and there is indeed merit to it. Expressions such as "trust your gut" and "gut instinct" refer to this undefinable inner intuitive detection system.

Inner strength is your core. See if you can feel your physical inner strength while performing daily activities such as mowing that huge lawn (some days it seems huge even if it isn't), raking seemingly endless piles of leaves, and vacuuming the carpet. All of these activities can strengthen your core. (We often recommend finding a 1970s thick shag carpet for our advanced core-strengthening vacuuming program.) Seriously though, have fun noticing, acknowledging, and being thankful for your core strength with every twist and turn. As you lift your child, open a jar of peanut butter, or pet the dog, notice how your core stabilizes your movement.

Now imagine all aspects of throwing a ball. See it first in your mind, then enact it physically in slow motion, feeling the origin of your movement. Notice that your energy moves through your shoulder, elbow, and wrist, finally releasing the ball from your hand, the end of the power chain. Your legs are the beginning of your power, working in conjunction with your core engine (your abs) to generate force outward through your torso and arm until you release the ball from your hand at the optimal peak of energy flow. This is the same action and knowledge that a martial artist uses when lowering her center of gravity and bending her knees to deliver a commanding punch. A boxer who arm-punches can never knock out his opponent. A knockout punch begins from the foot; power is generated up through the knee, hip, core, shoulder, and arm and ultimately explodes through the fist. Applying this knowledge to your golf swing, tennis swing, bat swing, throw, stride, stroke, kick, jab, or brick-breaking skills will give them new speed and power, allow you to exert less energy, and improve your overall endurance . . . and your jump shot will be the envy of the court.

Core muscles will always be stronger when trained as a single functional unit. Strengthening core muscles with only machine weights and crunches seldom elicits great results. Bodybuilders isolate muscle groups for definition, while other athletes train their stabilizers for function. Stabilizers keep you balanced and are synergists. Sprinters offer a great example of how core strength affects function. A sprinter who trains only the legs will not be as strong as a sprinter who trains the core and upper body as well. Sprinters who do not train their upper bodies cannot run as fast, and if their core is weak, the power chain between the arms and legs is broken. If you watch a sprinter closely, especially in slow motion, you can see the amazing role that abdominal muscles play. Great sprinters employ long, extended strides; exhibit ever-present stability in their core; balance the center; and maximize the coordinated movement of the arms and legs.

Inner strength, motivation, and inspiration are the essence of your core and the beginning of any enjoyable exercise experience, including ab training. Put your mind into your core. Be aware of your body in space. This kinesthetic awareness not only prevents accidents and injury but allows you to perform at your highest level. Gymnasts are a beautiful example of kinesthetic awareness. Extending, rotating, spinning, landing, balancing, releasing, and showcasing strength moves, gymnasts learn to be aware of their bodies, trusting and using their core instincts and strength at all times.

Functioning, flexible abdominal muscles constantly stabilize, working as a unit to protect your core. You can move with increased balance and body control if your midsection is strong enough to steady your movement. Flexibility is apparent in great athletes (such as Michael Jordan, Michelle Kwan, Karch Kiraly, Marion Jones), creating strong, resilient grace that is such a joy to behold. A tense or tight athlete seldom triumphs over a flexible, core-trained athlete, unless the competition involves pulling a Sherman tank with his teeth.

Overall quickness and speed also improve as you naturally strengthen your core. The abdominals act as a potentially powerful liaison between the upper and lower body, so that you will indeed experience more speed as your abs get stronger. Athletes such as gymnasts, martial artists, football players, soccer players, volleyball players, and basketball players develop strong abs naturally through their many drills and exercises. Remember that Bruce Lee did not rely on the latest ab contraption to strengthen his core. Multidimensional martial training produced quite an amazing set of abs. All athletes use their cores as a single stabilizing unit in their sports. A synergistic relationship exists between speed and strength in developing core power. Increasing speed through sports training or increasing strength through the exercises in this book will increase power. And a powerful core enhances your sport and your life.

Every movement you make begins from your core. The core includes muscles that surround the stomach and lower back area (see illustration). These are the pelvic floor muscles, the external obliques (visible through the skin as the "hands in the front pocket" muscles), the internal obliques (under the external obliques, shaped like an upside-down V), the rectus abdominis (the "six-pack"), the multifidus (the Christmas-tree-shaped muscle in the lower back), the erector spinae (which run adjacent to the spine from the sacrum to the skull), and the transversus abdominis (which acts almost like a weight belt because it contracts when you bear down, cough, or sneeze). If these muscles aren't strong and supple, you won't perform your best in sport or physical activity, and even sneezing will be a pain.

Strengthening the core stabilizes the pelvis. The pelvis stabilizes the hip. The hip stabilizes the foot. Like a pebble dropped into a pond, the effects of the core are felt throughout the whole body. A shoulder problem may be caused by the inflexibility of the abdominal muscles. Although the upper portion of the abs may be strong from hundreds of daily crunches, the entire rectus abdominis may be tight from performing crunches on the floor. Soon after the abdominals are stretched on a device such as a stability ball or in a standing yoga sun salutation pose, flexibility will improve, and the shoulder problem may disappear.

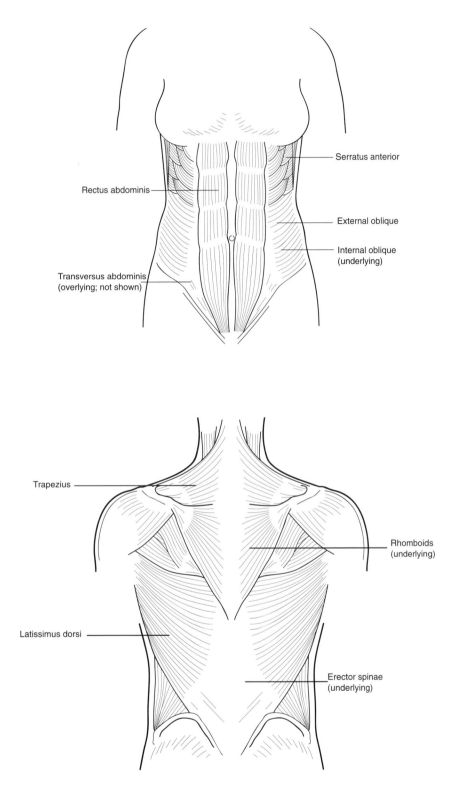

Rectus abdominis

Serratus anterior

External oblique

Internal oblique
(underlying)

Transversus abdominis
(overlying; not shown)

Trapezius

Rhomboids
(underlying)

Latissimus dorsi

Erector spinae
(underlying)

All movements begin from the core muscles.

It is important to prepare the torso for flexion (leaning forward), extension (leaning backward), and rotation (turning sideways) by training the abs, back, and obliques. The core inner muscles are the lower back muscles, gluteals, and diaphragm. These are also the posture muscles. The outer muscles are the superficial muscles of the spine and abdomen. The inner and outer units work together to create fluid, controlled, and powerful action.

Muscles in the abdomen are responsible for maintaining posture in all situations. A strong midline prevents injury, allowing you to move in a variety of angles, changing direction instantaneously and feeling more secure in all movements. But depending on the activity, the center of gravity changes. For example, your center of gravity is outside your body during a jump. Your center of gravity changes again when your feet touch ground and again when you turn to run. A stable, well-trained core enables you to seamlessly perform all these moves with maximum strength and flexibility.

## Inside the Muscle

There are two basic types of muscle fibers in the abdominal area: type I and type II. During 10 repetitions of crunches, the first several repetitions use primarily type I oxidative fibers, then type IIa intermediate fibers are recruited, and finally type IIb nonoxidative fibers push out that last rep.

Type I (slow-twitch) fibers are red endurance fibers and make up the postural muscles. Muscles made of type I fibers hold the body erect. Type I fibers are recruited first. Although they are capable of less force, they can perform more repetitions than type II fibers. Type I fibers are aerobic (oxidative). They are smaller and contain less glycogen than type II fibers, but their myoglobin content is high. Type I fibers use an oxygen-based process for energy, so they can store more oxygen than type II fibers. Type I fibers also have a higher capillary density than type II fibers.

Type II (fast-twitch) fibers are recruited for fast, powerful moves such as medicine ball twists. There are two subclasses of type II fibers. Type IIa intermediate fibers are somewhat oxidative and use a combination of aerobic and glycogen systems. These are recruited after type I fibers. Type IIa fibers have moderate myoglobin content, capillary density, force production, and endurance.

Type IIb fibers are anaerobic (nonoxidative). They are stronger and provide more force but fatigue quickly. Type IIb fibers have a high glycogen content and a fast twitch rate. They have few capillaries and low endurance but a high power output.

The number and type (fast-twitch or slow-twitch) of muscle fibers in the body is determined during the second trimester of a fetus's development. Each abdominal muscle fiber is 75 percent water, 20 percent protein, and 5 percent phosphates, calcium, magnesium, sodium, potassium, chloride, fats, carbohydrates, and amino acids.

Let's talk briefly about muscular endurance. Executing 100 crunches is quite a feat for most people, but contracting the abdominals continuously for 30 seconds is a different activity entirely. Between each crunch people typically rest their abdominal muscles, relaxing the contraction briefly. An isometric contraction held for 30 seconds can be difficult unless you train your abs correctly (make sure to breathe when you hold a contraction). This ability to sustain a contraction is called muscular endurance.

Sustaining a push-up position in perfect body alignment also requires core stability and muscular endurance. When you stand in an upright position for a prolonged period of time, the more stability and endurance you have in your abdominal muscles, the better your posture and the less prone your lower back will be to slipping into a precarious and potentially injurious position. Keep in mind that both strength and endurance are important when developing your abs.

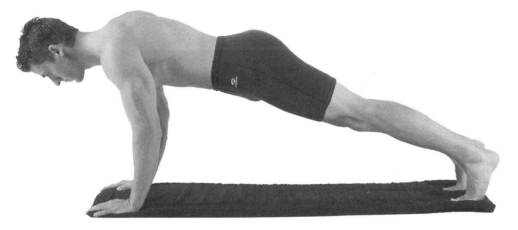

A perfectly sustained push-up position is a demonstration of core stability and muscular endurance.

## BENEFITS OF DEVELOPING THE CORE

Improving the core offers many benefits, but we focus on six major benefits: core control, balance, strength, endurance, power, and speed.

- **Core control.** Imagine a piece of string tied around your waist at all times. This imaginary string should not be broken during any movement. This requires that you maintain a constant contraction of your abdominal muscles, especially your transversus abdominis.
- **Proprioception (balance).** Can you keep your balance while kneeling on a stability ball? After training for a month on this program, you should notice a significant improvement in your balance. Check your balance by standing on one leg with the other foot off the floor. Hold for 30

seconds. Try the other leg. Now close your eyes. Open your eyes and continue standing on one leg while you toss a ball of your choice back and forth to a partner. Now recite the Gettysburg Address (just kidding).

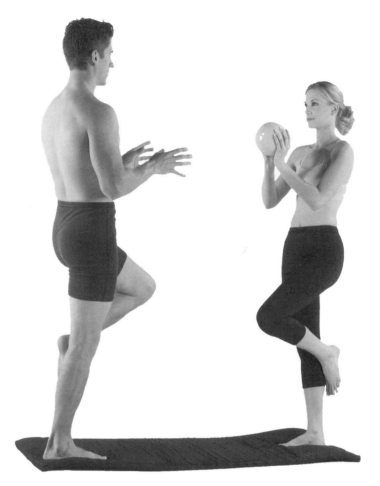

Core training improves balance. Try this quick test to find out where you stand: Stand on one leg while passing a ball to your partner.

• **Strength.** Our program strengthens the entire core so that every activity is easier and more efficient. The pool exercises and dynamic strength exercises using your own body weight as resistance require that you generate strength from your core.

• **Endurance.** You may not know it, but standing, walking, or any movement involves core muscular endurance. Core muscular endurance can be developed while waiting in line or sitting on an airplane. It is all about learning to contract the abdominals isometrically. Press your lower back into your chair by contracting your abdominal muscles. Hold for 10 seconds. Add 2 seconds a week until you can maintain a core contraction for 30 seconds (or until you wear out the fabric of the chair).

• **Power.** After you have improved your endurance, control, balance, and dynamic strength, it is time to work on power. Even if you do not consider yourself an athlete, a powerful core will help you sprint, carry a suitcase, or sprint while carrying a suitcase. Our plyometric training will develop your core power.

- **Speed.** The reason many of our exercises begin slowly and speed up with progression is that people who always move slowly in training move slowly in performance too. That is why it is advisable to train at different speeds. Your performance improvement depends on how you train. If you always move slowly, what happens when you must sprint to a bus? Either you injure yourself or you miss the bus.

## BEGINNING THE PROGRAM

Well, you have certainly not missed the bus, even though you may have been on the wrong bus for a while, dabbling in the so-called "magic bullets" of fitness. Release all preconceptions; we all have to learn at some point that quick fixes don't work and that great results are achieved by smart training. Our training is the quickest, safest way to great abs and a strong core. The process is up to you, though, and your seat on the bus is guaranteed as long as you participate. Train in the morning or at night, on your lunch break or at home. In our program, you can tackle strength, flexibility, and core stability all at once.

The benefits of exercise are awesome if your body is ready to train. But working out is stressful, and if your body has an ailment, adding stress can be debilitating. If you are over 40 years old, get a physical exam before you begin ab training. If you have an ache or pain that doesn't go away after a week, see a physician. "No pain is sane"—that's our motto.

Women are generally more flexible than men, but they may not be as strong, at least at first. Therefore, women should take the following precautions:

- Be careful not to hyperextend a joint, especially during pregnancy.
- Avoid competing with your male counterpart on strength moves.
- Don't be afraid to take an extra day off between training sessions. Women often require more rest than men, theoretically because they lack testosterone.

Men are generally cockier than women (because of testosterone and big egos) and tend to overtrain, not feeling the effects of their workouts or trying too hard too fast. Therefore, men should take the following precautions:

- Slow down.
- Have patience with yourself.
- Stretch at the end of your workout.

We hope that everyone reads the tips for both men and women because each person is unique and all tips really apply to everyone (except that men don't need to worry about special precautions during pregnancy). You should also eat properly for sustenance and to further empower your workouts. We do not believe in the use of steroids or physique-enhancing supplements. True bodybuilding is done with natural foods and without drugs.

# 2

# STRETCHING TO STRENGTHEN:
## Key Flexibility Exercises

Ever wonder why a 100-pound ballet dancer has exquisitely refined calf muscles but many 200-pound bodybuilders who lift the heaviest weights can't get cut calves? The key is flexibility in plantar flexion, the point and flex of the foot. A ballet dancer flexes and points with natural body-weight resistance, over time developing the muscles to their maximum potential. An inflexible bodybuilder, who has limited range of motion and uses too much weight, wastes training time, risks injury, and achieves limited results. Flexibility of the abdominals is as significant as strength. If your abdominals are not flexible, you not only limit potential muscular development through lack of range of motion, but you also risk injury. Flexibility and strength through a broader range of motion is the desired goal for those seeking athletic abs.

This training program employs what we call flexible strength. This means that when you are lying down, your spine is in a natural arch or neutral position before you begin core exercises. This improves core flexibility and increases muscle strength. Strength within a broader range of motion (flexibility) is the goal. For the muscle fibers to contract fully, they should be prestretched to about 1.2 times their normal resting length. This initial stretch allows more crossbridging of muscle fibers to get a greater contraction. The antagonist muscle should be relaxed and flexible when the agonist is contracting for maximum strength and power. In optimal training, there is a strong relationship between strength and stretch.

All human movements have a strength and stretch component. As one side stretches (abs), the other side contracts (lower and middle back), and vice versa. From yoga's sun salutation (stretching the abs, opening the chest and shoulders) to chi kung's bending bear (lengthening the entire back and hamstrings), and other simple, easy-to-follow muscle-lengthening exercises, our program illustrates the symbiotic relationship between the abdominal and back muscles. This symbiotic relationship between opposing muscle groups is yet another reason to balance your training.

Limited-range crunches shorten the rectus abdominis muscle. If you are not stretching your abs or training your lower back (the opposing muscle group) in conjunction with your ab training, the torso will eventually pull forward from lack of flexibility, eliciting a muscular postural imbalance. The bottom line is that the more muscularly balanced and flexible your torso is, the more comfortable you will be, the more efficient your movement will be, and the less chance you will have of injury.

Imbalanced strength has a ripple effect. Try this experiment. Lie on your back. Raise your right leg toward the ceiling until you feel a stretch in your hamstring. Hold that stretch and note the angle of your leg in reference to your body.

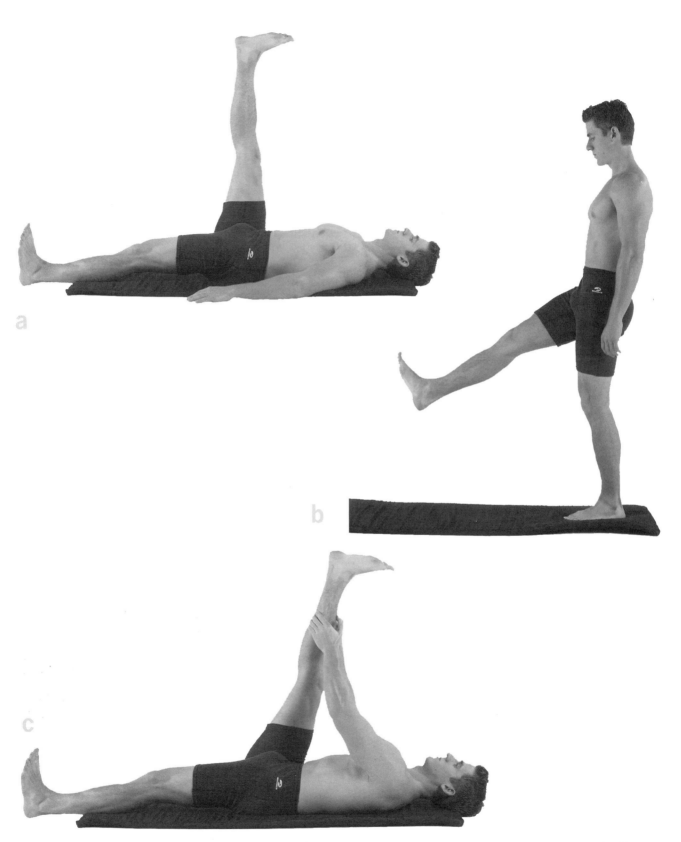

(a) First, lie on your back and note the angle of your leg in reference to your body as you hold the hamstring stretch. (b) Second, how high can you raise your leg while standing? Compare the angle of your leg in the standing stretch to the angle you achieved while lying on your back. (c) Third, lie on the floor again. This time use your hands to stretch your leg further.

Now stand. Raise your right leg again, lifting in front, knee toward the ceiling. How far could you lift it? Why couldn't you raise your leg to the same angle as when you were lying on the floor? Try another experiment. Lie on your back and raise your leg as you did before. This time, grasp your leg and slowly add a few inches to your previous stretch until you feel a slight discomfort in your hamstring.

Release your grip and attempt to hold your leg in your newfound extended stretch. When you first perform this experiment, it is typical for the leg to bounce back down about 30 degrees. Our goal is to eliminate that 30-degree drop. Obviously, the hamstring was flexible enough to extend that extra 30 degrees in the first place, but the hands needed to help pull the leg into position. Why couldn't the leg stay in the extended stretch without help from the hands? The answer to this question is that the leg is just not strong enough (though you may or may not believe it when you look into a mirror). Your leg dropped 30 degrees due to a lack of muscle strength and stability. The antagonist muscles to your hamstrings are your quadriceps and hip flexors. These muscles, along with your core, must be extremely strong to hold your hamstrings in a lengthened stretch, especially against the pull of gravity.

Bodybuilders sport well-defined muscles, while aerobicizers have small waistlines. Swimmers and runners possess incredible endurance. Flexibility is a common denominator in beautiful physiques and long-lived sport performances. Plus, when you need some validation, you can contort for your friends at parties, squeeze into glass boxes, or join the circus.

## Balance

Proprioception is different from the balance that comes from the semicircular canals in the inner ear. Proprioceptors are special nerves that provide the brain with feedback about where the body is in space. The pelvis has the highest concentration of proprioceptors in the entire body. As you train your core, you stimulate these proprioceptors, thus improving your balance and mobility.

If you neglect core training and do not improve your balance, your ability to balance will soon diminish. Balance helps all aspects of sports performance. Good balance also helps you break a fall and minimize injury.

Core training improves proprioception, which equals balance. Enough said.

# FLEXIBILITY AND RELAXATION

Flexibility exercises take only a relaxed few minutes (but don't say, "I'm in a hurry; I've got to stretch") and require no special equipment. When we in the fitness industry talk shop, we are all amazed at the number of students who ignore their flexibility or painfully rush through their flexibility exercises. A stretching and relaxation program improves posture and sport performance. Stretching maintains joints and prevents low-back and other injuries. Stretching is also a relaxing method of mental preparation before (and after) training. We have some great stretching and relaxation techniques inspired by yoga and tai chi and some stretches highlighting each muscle group. This way you can work both sides of your brain as well as your body. We recommend a light walk, our yoga/tai chi warm-up, and our full-body stretching sequence prior to a workout. Feel free to lengthen and stretch throughout the day to keep your body active and energized.

A slow, continuous stretch is desired—no bouncing. Really settle into the stretch. Relax and breathe—remember, breath is life. Inhalation is the preparation, exhalation is the release. Feel the beauty of releasing tension as you move into each stretched position, breathing normally, easing further if desired on another relaxed exhalation. Hold the stretch (but not your breath) at the limits of joint motion until you feel tension in your muscle, then relax. Go for comfort. Soft music in the background is nice. Stretch without a teeth-clenched, red-ballooned face (it's just not pretty). Relax your neck and your shoulders, and notice where your body carries tension, self-monitoring your joints, muscles, and tendons. In tai chi, we talk about the "spider in the web." Your spider is centered at your dan tien (core, below your navel), while your web is your entire body. Perform an internal inventory of your body as you relax into your stretching. No pain is gain. Settle into your pose like a yogi, breathing and expanding, shifting your energy slowly down into your center core, out of your chest, neck, and throat. Your body will adapt, and soon you will be stretching comfortably.

# Key Points for the Perfect Stretch

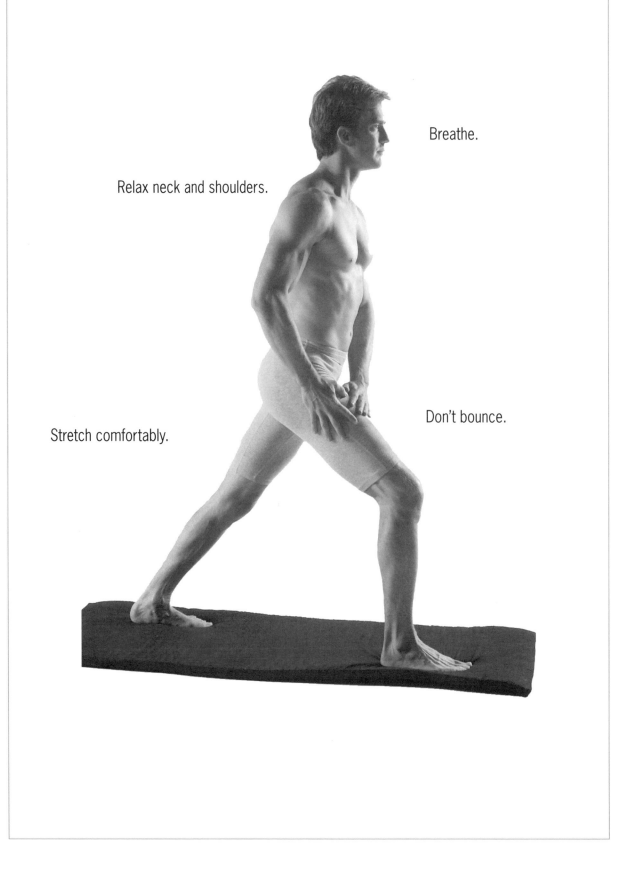

Breathe.

Relax neck and shoulders.

Don't bounce.

Stretch comfortably.

This is a combination of ancient Chinese chi kung moves. Stand comfortably, joints relaxed. Tap your body all over as if waking up the skin. As you tap each arm inside and out, each leg inside and out, the outer thighs, the inner thighs, buttocks, abs, lower back, shoulders, head, neck, face, everything, you will feel the relaxation and preparation going deeper into the muscles as well. As you feel this, start to relax your joints, gently shaking out the tension (think of Elvis), dropping your chin forward slightly to relax the neck, bending slightly in the waist to loosen the lower back, and so on. Anything goes, so have fun and make it comfortable for yourself.

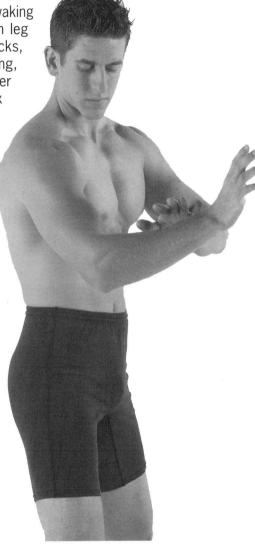

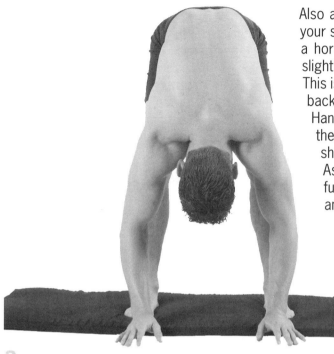

Also an ancient chi kung move, the bending bear prepares your spine and lower back for exercise quite nicely. Stand in a horse stance: feet parallel, shoulder-width apart, knees slightly bent. Bend forward slowly, one vertebra at a time (a). This is a great lesson in working with gravity, opening up the back of the body, and learning to release tension naturally. Hang there for a little while, legs stabilized, breathing out the tension; notice how it takes a few seconds to relax the shoulders, head, neck, arms, hands, fingers, and torso. As you breathe, feel free to vocalize your exhalations, further releasing tension in your abdomen, lower back, and legs.

a

Once you feel completely relaxed, slowly roll up, one vertebra at a time, feeling your body stretch naturally with the help of gravity. Now repeat the same process leaning your torso over your right leg (b), rolling up slowly again, and then over your left leg, keeping your weight centered. If it doesn't feel like heaven, do it again and learn to let go. About 30 seconds for each stage of bending bear is appropriate.

b

This modified yoga pose is great for relaxing the chest, neck, face, shoulders, and abs and for energizing the heart and lungs (pretty vital). It also just downright feels good. Stand with your feet slightly apart for balance. Place your hands (fingertips toward the ground) in the small of your back for support. Inhale as you expand, lifting your breastbone up toward the sky. Exhale as you relax back into an open chest and core stretch, elbows gently pulling in toward each other behind you. Continue breathing as you feel your head slowly tilting back, stretching your neck, relaxing your jaw, feeling the comfort of the pose as you keep your breastbone lifted. Remember to keep the upwardly expansive feeling, relying on gravity to stretch you into a natural arch of the back. Enjoy each magnificent breath. Feel free to reposition your hands and feet; repeat the pose if you like.

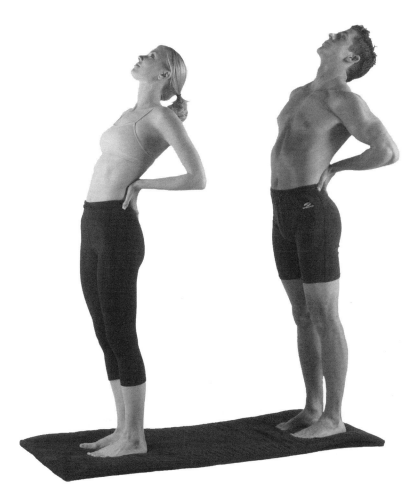

If we were marooned on a desert island with angry natives who allowed us only one relaxation pose per day, this would be our choice. Also known as the baby pose or infant pose, the child's pose can be adapted for all levels of flexibility. Start on all fours. Ease your way back, buttocks to heels, resting your forehead on the floor. Your arms, hands, and fingers are relaxed by your sides (a). If this is difficult for you, keep your elbows forward, resting your head on your hands (b). You can also use pillows under your feet or shins or behind your knees until you develop more flexibility. While in the pose, breathe, relax your head and neck, and feel your lower back expanding and relaxing. Set goals, meditate, feel your circulation and life force. The child's pose really clears the mind, relieves tension in the stomach, and is great at the beginning or end of the day.

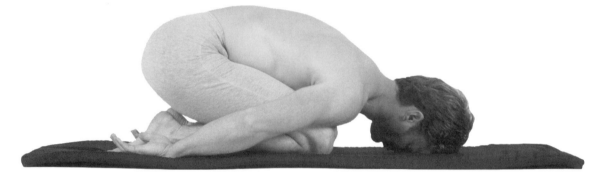

a

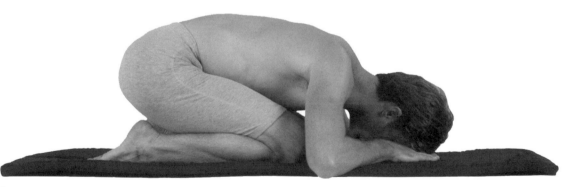

b

# STRETCHING SEQUENCE

Now that your body and mind are relaxed and energized, it is time to embark on a complete and specific full-body stretching sequence. Take your time for all of the stretches; do not rush. (It is best not to rush anything, for that matter.) Keep in mind that you are creating better body awareness and muscle memory each time you go through the full-body stretching sequence. Make this sequence so familiar that your body feels what to do next and your mind can relax. Be mindful of your muscles throughout each and every exercise to achieve your best performance. Breathe calmly at the edge of discomfort as you execute each move. Realize that you will improve and that this is the perfect routine for you today.

If you do not have time to do the entire stretching routine, choose the stretches that you enjoy most or the stretches that focus on your specific needs, for example, sport preparation or a target muscle group. It is advisable, however, to stretch your entire body to achieve a balance of strength and flexibility.

Combining proprioceptive neuromuscular facilitation (PNF) and active isolated (AI) stretching is a magnificent way to improve flexibility and performance. To perform these exercises, you first contract your agonist (the muscle you are trying to stretch) for three seconds. You then relax and stretch that same muscle for three seconds. Next you contract your antagonist (the opposite muscle) for three seconds, then relax and stretch the agonist muscle again for three seconds. Relax. Although it sounds complicated, remember that you are dealing with only two muscle groups at a time and stretching only one (the agonist) in each set. Using the biceps and triceps as an example, we can break the sequence down like this:

1. Contract agonist (biceps).
2. Stretch agonist (biceps).
3. Contract antagonist (triceps).
4. Stretch agonist (biceps).

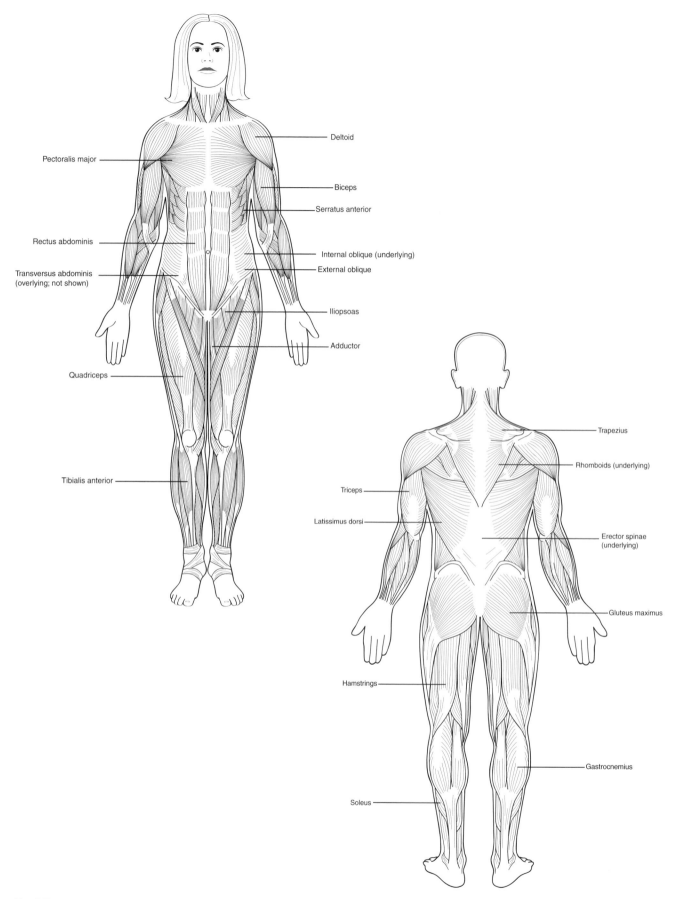

Deltoid

Pectoralis major

Biceps

Serratus anterior

Rectus abdominis

Internal oblique (underlying)

External oblique

Transversus abdominis
(overlying; not shown)

Iliopsoas

Adductor

Quadriceps

Tibialis anterior

Trapezius

Rhomboids (underlying)

Triceps

Latissimus dorsi

Erector spinae
(underlying)

Gluteus maximus

Hamstrings

Gastrocnemius

Soleus

Flexibility is an important part of muscle development. Learn the muscles of your body and treat them right.

Stand and bend slightly at the waist. Place your hands on your thighs while you extend your right foot forward. Drop your hips back and lean your chest toward your right knee until you feel a light stretch in your hamstrings. Contract your hamstrings for three seconds by pressing your right heel into the floor. Relax and stretch a little bit further by drawing your hips back. Contract your thigh muscles (quadriceps) for three seconds. Relax and stretch your hamstrings a little bit further. Hold for three seconds. Switch legs and repeat.

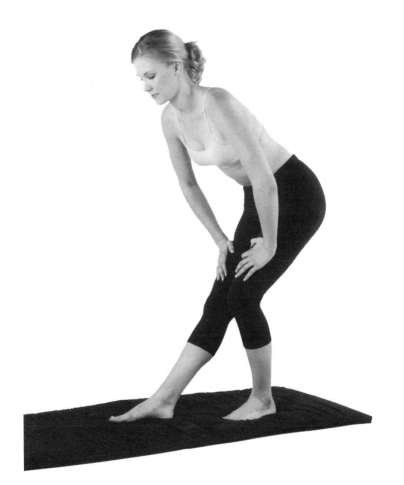

# LUNGE (HIP FLEXORS)

Take a step forward as if you were about to perform a lunge. Hold that position as you tilt your pelvis forward so you feel a stretch in your hip flexor (iliopsoas) of your back leg. Contract your hip flexor for three seconds. Relax and stretch your hip flexor. Contract your gluteal muscles by pressing your back heel into the floor for three seconds. Relax and stretch your hip flexor a bit further. Stop when you feel tension. Hold for three seconds. Switch legs and repeat.

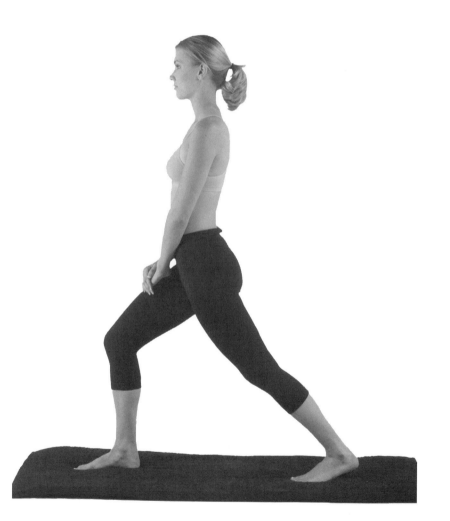

To stretch your calf muscles, assume a lunge position. Keep your back heel on the floor and your back leg almost completely straight as you lean into the lunge. You should feel the stretch in the back of your back leg. Contract your calf muscle for three seconds by pressing the ball of your back foot into the floor. Relax and stretch your calf muscles a bit further. Contract your shin muscle (tibialis anterior) by lifting the toes of your back foot toward the ceiling. Hold for three seconds. Relax and stretch your calf muscles a bit further. Stop when you feel tension. Hold for three seconds. Switch legs and repeat.

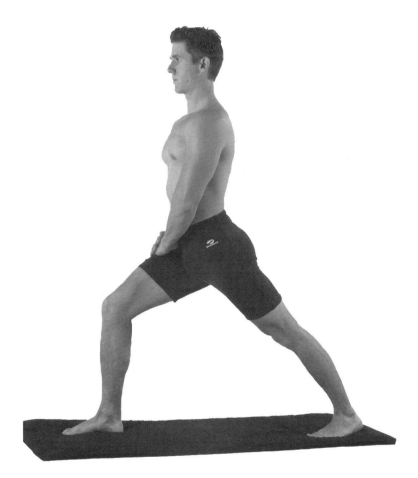

STRETCHING TO STRENGTHEN: Key Flexibility Exercises

# INNER-CALF STRETCH (SOLEUS)

To stretch the muscle underneath your calf, assume a lunge position. This time, instead of holding your back leg straight, bend it until you feel a stretch in your lower leg. Stop when you feel tension. Now contract your soleus by keeping your knee bent and pressing the ball of your back foot into the floor for three seconds. Relax and stretch your soleus a bit further. Contract your shin muscle (tibialis anterior) by lifting the toes of your back foot toward the ceiling. Hold for three seconds. Relax and stretch your soleus until you feel tension. Hold for three seconds. Switch legs and repeat.

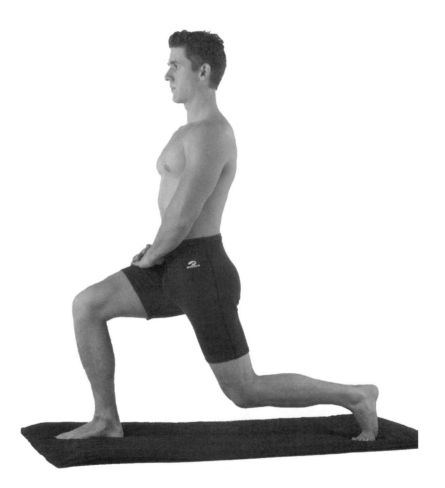

# STANDING THIGH STRETCH (QUADRICEPS)

For balance, hold onto a chair with your right hand and bend your left knee so that you almost kick yourself in the butt. Grab the top of your left foot with your left hand. Gently pull your heel toward your butt with your left hand. Stop when you feel tension. Contract your quadriceps muscle for three seconds. Relax. Stretch your quads a little further. Contract your hamstrings for three seconds. Relax and stretch your quads until you feel tension. Hold for three seconds. Switch legs and repeat.

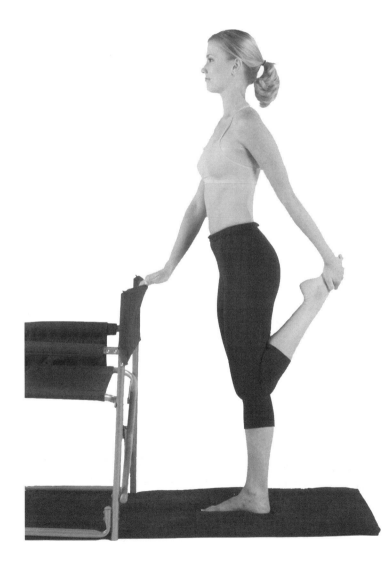

# LATERAL LEG STRETCH (ABDUCTORS)

This is a stretch for the leg abductors and iliotibial band. Stand sideways behind a chair. Place your right hand on the back of the chair. Slowly lean your right hip toward the chair until you feel tension in your right hip abductors. Contract your abductors for three seconds. Relax and stretch your abductors. Contract your adductors for three seconds. Relax. Stretch your abductors by leaning a little closer to the chair. Hold for three seconds. Switch sides and repeat.

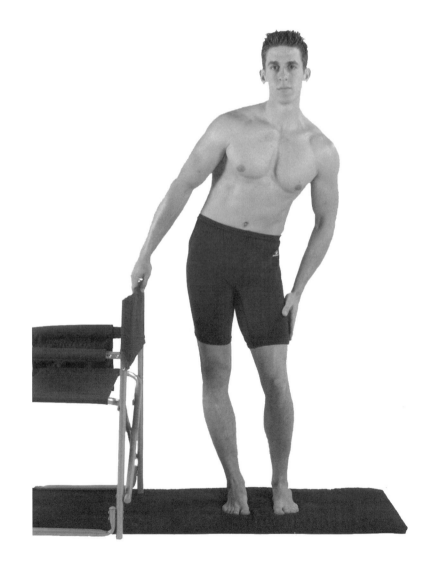

# KNEELING CHEST STRETCH (PECTORALS)

Kneel in front of a chair, facing the chair. Extend your arms and place your hands on the seat with your elbows slightly bent. Slowly drop your chest toward the floor until you feel a stretch in your chest (pectoral muscles). Contract your pectoral muscles for three seconds. Relax and stretch your pectorals again. Then contract your rhomboids by retracting your shoulder blades for three seconds. Relax and stretch your pectorals a bit further. Stop when you feel tension. Hold for three seconds. Repeat.

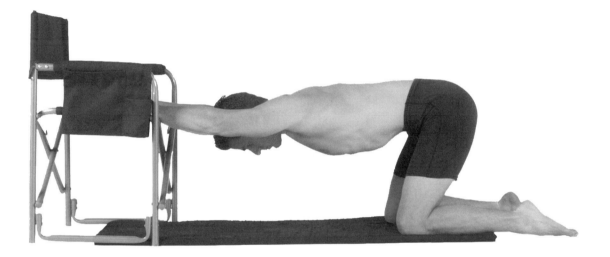

Stand and reach up as high as you can with both arms over your head. Look at your hands. Feel the stretch in your upper back. Contract those same back muscles for three seconds. Relax. Stretch a little higher. Contract your chest and abdominal muscles for three seconds. Relax and stretch a bit higher. Stop when you feel tension. Hold for three seconds.

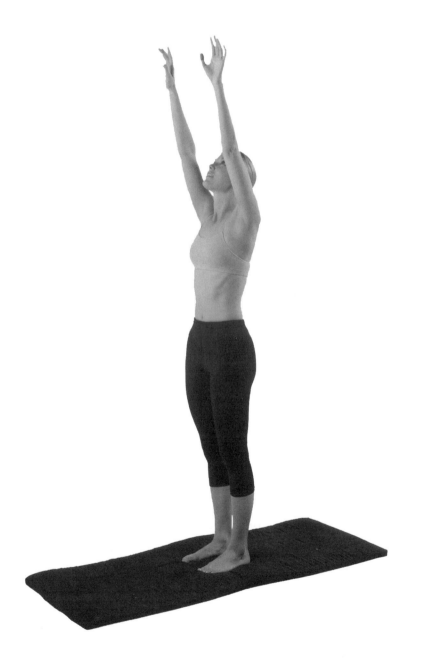

Stand and reach up toward the ceiling with both arms. Place your left hand on your right elbow, pulling your right hand down your back. Stop when you feel tension. Contract the muscles in the back of your right arm (triceps) for three seconds. Relax and stretch a bit further. Contract your right biceps for three seconds. Relax and stretch your right triceps a bit further. Hold for three seconds. Switch sides and repeat.

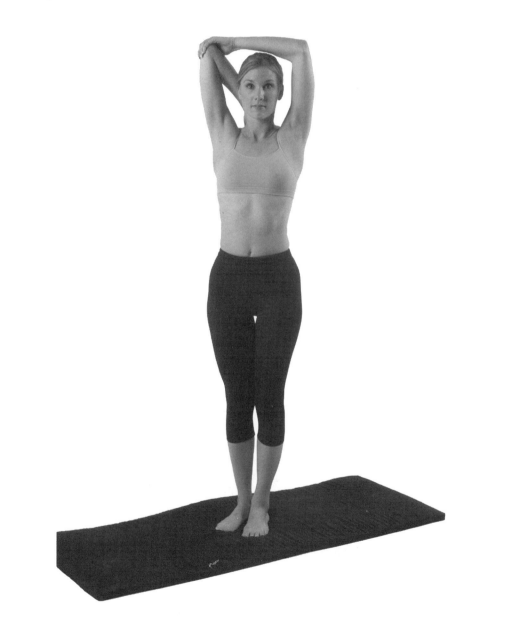

# SHOULDER STRETCH (DELTOIDS)

Stand and grab your right elbow with your left hand and pull it across your body. Stop when you feel tension in your shoulder (lateral deltoid). Contract that muscle for three seconds. Relax and stretch a bit further. Contract your pectoral for three seconds. Relax and stretch your right lateral deltoid one more time. Hold for three seconds. Switch sides and repeat.

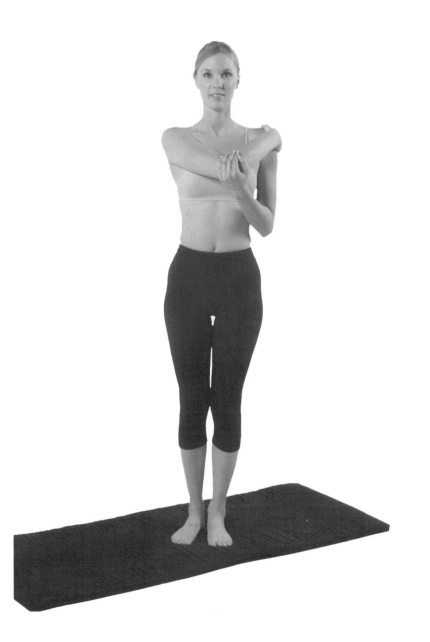

Stand comfortably and bring your chin toward your chest (a). Contract the muscles in the back of your neck. Relax and stretch a bit further. Then contract the muscles in the front of your neck. Relax and stretch. Drop your head back slightly, lifting your chin toward the ceiling. Relax and stretch a bit further. Then bring your right ear toward your right shoulder (b). Contract the muscles in the right side of your neck. Relax them and stretch a bit further. Contract the muscles in the left side of your neck. Relax and stretch toward your right side again. Then bring your left ear toward your left shoulder. Contract the muscles in the left side of your neck. Relax them and stretch a bit further. Contract the muscles in the right side of your neck. Relax and stretch toward your left side again.

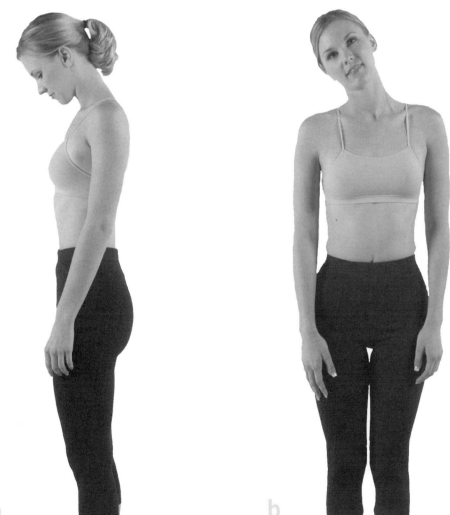

a                                           b

---

STRETCHING TO STRENGTHEN: Key Flexibility Exercises

# FULL-BODY STRETCH

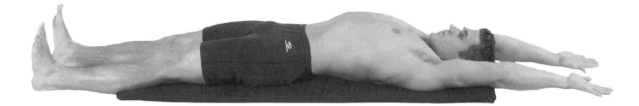

Lie on your back and stretch as tall as you can. Reach as high over your head as you can and extend your heels as far as you can in the other direction. Contract all of the muscles in the front of your body. Relax and reach higher. Contract all of the muscles in the back of your body. Relax and reach higher. Hold for three seconds. Relax.

# SUPINE HIP FLEXOR STRETCH (ILIOPSOAS)

Lie down on your back and brace yourself with your left hand. Keep your left leg extended; pull your right knee toward your chest. Reach behind your right knee with your right hand and pull your right knee closer to your chest. Stop when you feel tension. Contract your hip flexor to raise your knee even higher. Relax and stretch a bit further. Then contract your hamstrings by pressing against your arm for three seconds. Relax and stretch your hip flexor a bit further. Hold for three seconds. Switch sides and repeat.

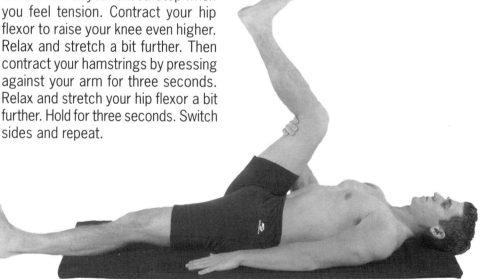

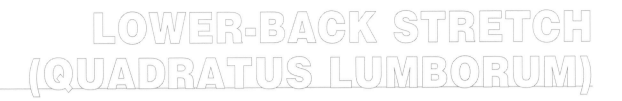

Lie on your back. Bring both knees toward your chest and place your arms around your knees to stretch your lower back. Contract your hip flexors and quadriceps and bring your knees closer to your chest. Relax and hold the stretch. Now contract your hamstrings and gluteals against your arms for three seconds. Relax and try to bring your knees even closer to your chest. Hold for three seconds. Relax.

# BUTTOCKS STRETCH
# (GLUTEALS)

Lie on your back. Extend your left leg and keep your left heel on the floor. Point your right foot high toward the ceiling so that your legs form a 90-degree angle. Slowly lower your right foot to the left so that you feel a stretch in your right hip. As your leg crosses the midline of your body, gradually bend your right knee until it forms a 90-degree angle. Stop when you feel tension. Contract your right hip for three seconds. Relax and stretch a little bit further. Contract your right inner thigh (adductors) for three seconds. Relax and elongate the stretch; let gravity stretch your gluteals a bit further one more time. Hold for three seconds. Switch sides and repeat.

# WAIST STRETCH (OBLIQUES)

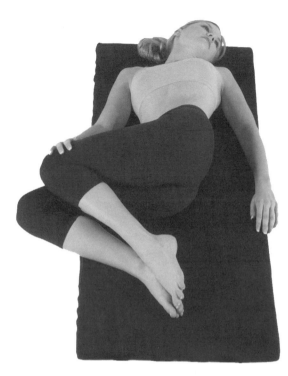

Lie on your back. Bring both knees toward your chest. Slowly lower your knees to the right as you look to your left. Feel the stretch in the side of your waist (your obliques). Stop when you feel tension. Contract those muscles for three seconds. Relax and stretch a bit further. Contract your opposite obliques for three seconds. Relax and increase your stretch. Switch sides and repeat.

# SITTING HAMSTRING STRETCH

Sit in a straddle position on the floor. Contract your right hamstring muscle. Hold the contraction for three seconds. Relax. Now exhale and bring your chest toward your right knee. Stop when you feel tension. Now contract your right quadriceps for three seconds. Relax and again bring your chest closer to your right knee. Hold for three seconds. Switch sides and repeat.

# STRADDLE LEG-ADDUCTOR STRETCH

Sit in a straddle position on the floor. Contract your hamstrings and your inner thigh muscles (adductors). Hold the contraction for three seconds. Relax. Now exhale and bring your chest toward the floor. Now contract your front thighs (quadriceps) and hip flexors for three seconds. Relax and stretch by bringing your chest closer to the floor. Stop when you feel tension. Hold for three seconds. Relax.

# SITTING GASTROCNEMIUS STRETCH

Sit on the floor. Place your right leg in front of you and hold it straight. Bend your left knee so that your foot stabilizes you on the floor. Reach toward the toes of your right foot with your right hand. If you can reach your toes, pull them back. Contract your calf muscle by pressing your toes against your fingers. Hold for three seconds. Relax. Exhale and stretch your calf muscles. Now contract your tibialis anterior by lifting your toes up toward your knee for three seconds. Relax and stretch your calf muscle a little bit further. Stop when you feel tension. Hold for three seconds. Switch sides and repeat.

Sit on the floor with your left leg straight and the sole of your right foot resting on the inside of the knee of your left leg. Bring your right foot across your knee and turn your upper body in the same direction. Feel the stretch in your torso (obliques). Contract your left oblique muscles and hold for three seconds. Relax and stretch a little bit further. Now contract your right oblique muscles for three seconds. Relax and stretch. Stop when you feel tension. Hold for three seconds. Switch sides and repeat.

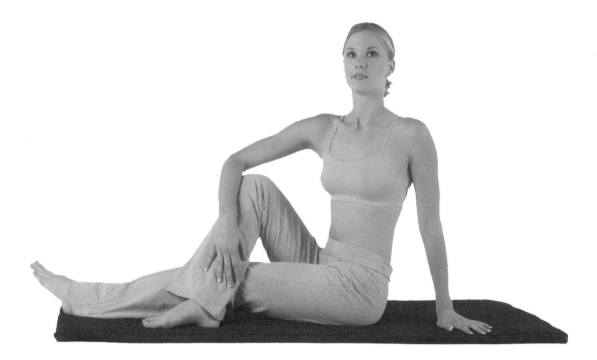

Sit on the floor with the soles of your feet together. Pull your feet as close to you as possible. Contract your inner thigh muscles (adductors) for three seconds. Relax. Exhale and stretch your adductors further. Now contract your gluteals for three seconds. Stop when you feel tension. Hold for three seconds. Relax.

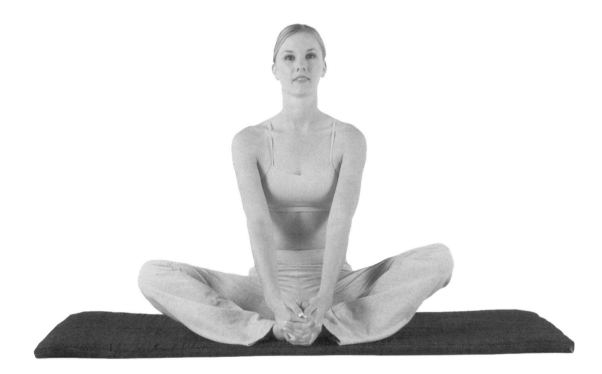

# SUPINE BUTTOCKS STRETCH

Lie on your back and place your left foot flat on the floor with the left knee bent. Place your right ankle across your left knee in a figure 4 position. Contract your hips and butt (gluteals) for three seconds. Relax. Exhale and stretch your gluteals a bit further by bringing your right foot toward your chest. Now contract the muscles of your inner thigh (adductors). Relax and see if you can bring your foot closer to your chest. Stop when you feel tension. Hold for three seconds. Switch sides and repeat.

# STANDING WAIST STRETCH (OBLIQUES)

Stand comfortably and interlock your fingers behind your head. Tilt your body sideways until you feel a stretch in your neck and your obliques. Contract those muscles for three seconds. Relax and stretch. Now contract the oblique muscles on the other side of your body for three seconds. Exhale and stretch a little bit further. Stop when you feel tension. Hold for three seconds. Switch sides and repeat.

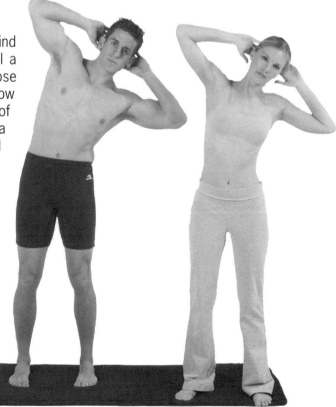

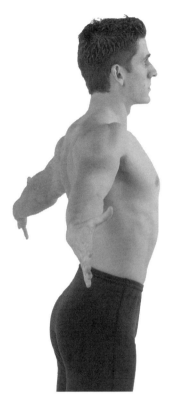

Stand with your feet shoulder-width apart. Stretch your arms out to your sides with your palms facing the ceiling. Slowly bring your arms back. Contract the muscles in your chest. Hold the contraction for three seconds. Relax. Exhale and stretch your pectorals a bit further by continuing to draw your arms backward. Now contract the muscles between your shoulder blades (rhomboids) for three seconds. Relax and see if you can move your arms back a bit further. Stop when you feel tension. Hold for three seconds. Relax.

# CORE STRETCH (ABDOMINALS)

Lie on your belly. Place your forearms under your chest with your palms on the floor. Press down with your hands until your elbows support you. Notice a stretch in your abdominal muscles. Contract your abdominals for three seconds. Exhale and stretch your abdominals a bit further by extending your elbows. Now contract your back muscles (erector spinae) and hold for three seconds. Relax. See if you can stretch a bit higher into spinal extension. Stop when you feel tension. Hold for three seconds. Relax.

Kneel on the floor on your hands and knees. Arch your back (a) and contract your upper and lower back muscles (erector spinae and multifidus) for three seconds. Exhale and round your back into a "cat-stretch" position (b). Now contract your abdominal muscles for three seconds. Relax and see if you can deepen your cat stretch. Stop when you feel tension. Hold for three seconds. Relax.

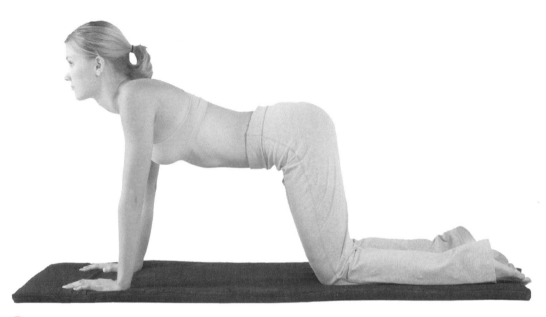

a

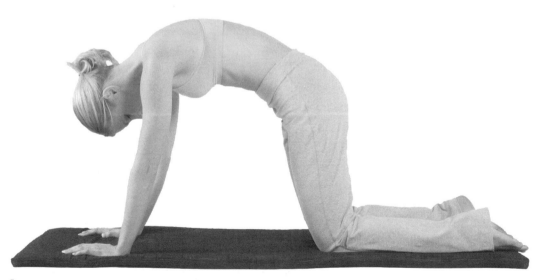

b

You can never have too many buttocks stretches. Lie on your back. Place your left foot on the floor with your knee bent. Place your right ankle across your left knee in a figure 4 position. Allow your right foot to pull your left knee to the right until you feel tension. Contract those muscles (gluteals, piriformis, and obliques). Hold the contraction for three seconds. Relax. Exhale and stretch a bit further. Now contract the antagonist muscles for three seconds: your ankle pulls against your knee as if you were performing an isometric tension exercise. Relax and see if you can stretch a bit further. Stop when you feel tension. Hold for three seconds. Switch sides and repeat.

# SPLIT INNER-THIGH STRETCH (ADDUCTORS)

Lie on your back. Extend your legs up and out in a split position until you feel a stretch in your inner-thigh muscles. Contract those adductor muscles for three seconds. Relax. Exhale and stretch a bit further. Now contract your abductors and gluteals for three seconds. Relax and see if your feet don't slide further down. Stop when you feel tension. Hold for three seconds. Relax.

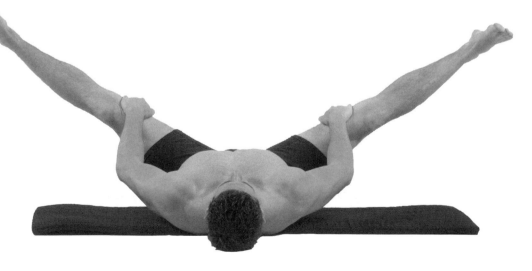

# SUPPORTED HIP-FLEXOR STRETCH

Face a wall and place both hands on it. Look over your left shoulder and slowly extend your left leg back until you feel tension in your hip flexor (a). Repeat with your right leg. Now turn your right side to the wall, and place your right hand on the wall. Look over your left shoulder and slowly extend your right leg to the side until you feel tension in your adductor muscles (b). Hold for three seconds. Turn your left side to the wall and repeat with your left leg.

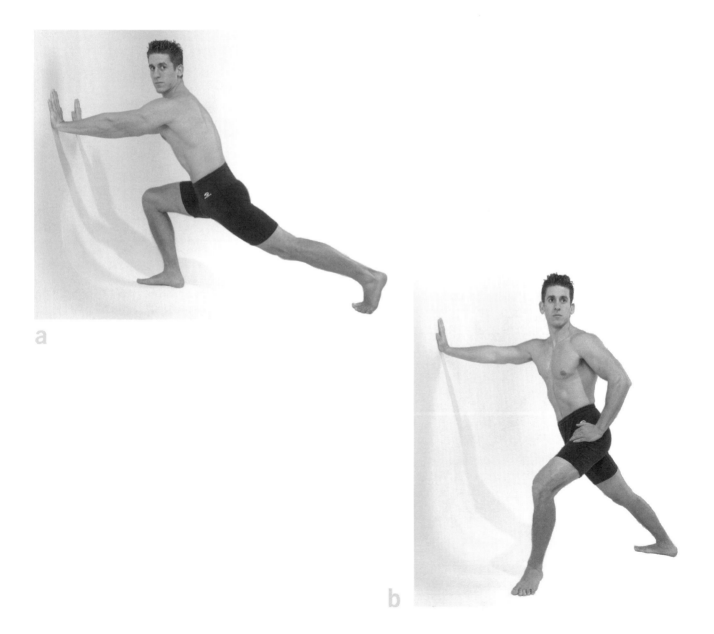

a

b

# 3

# BURNING OFF THE FAT:
## Cardio Training

As we have mentioned, 42 zillion crunches a day won't showcase your six-pack. However, pack in some great cardio interval training, a sensible eating plan, and our core drills, and behold, your six-pack takes form.

Cardio in the 1990s for some people often meant glancing longingly at the clock. For others though, it was a fun era of movement, expression, and dance. It is important to realize that each person is motivated in a different way. Some like the quiet of a treadmill, some like to cycle, and some like to dance till they drop. Enjoy yourself, but try not to go that far.

Cardio in this millennium can be quite varied, more customized to the individual. We know more now about fat-burning potential, and most experts (including us) recommend interval training, applying the knowledge that a person can burn more fat in a shorter period of time in interval training than in the traditional, sustained aerobic session of yesteryear.

Many aerobic instructors and participants learned that it is indeed the anaerobic (not sustained aerobic) bursts of energy that create the bodily changes of increased cardio endurance, lean muscle mass, and fat reduction. The music, the mood, and the rise and fall of energy in a traditional aerobics class created a natural, albeit accidental, interval-training class.

Many people have also discovered that a sustained activity such as running on a treadmill—although it greatly improves lung capacity and increases cardio output—seldom produces the noticeable physical changes that they desire. In fact, often the body actually stores fat to prepare for the sustained activity. Interval training innervates fast-twitch fibers and burns more calories than sustained aerobic activity. Even endurance athletes (distance swimmers, cyclists, and marathon runners) need a higher fat-to-muscle ratio to accomplish their task, and the body learns and responds to that (although in athletes this higher ratio does not show in the form of obesity). Even though marathon runners are always thin, their bodies are much different from the ripped, more muscular physiques of sprinters. You can also see the difference in the body of a short-distance swimmer versus a long-distance swimmer.

Interval training is simply the interspersing of work efforts with recovery cycles. Unlike workouts of sustained duration, interval exercises eventually work both aerobic and anaerobic systems, involve both slow- and fast-twitch muscle fibers, strengthen the heart, and burn fat in the safest, most efficient way. Start slowly and progress gradually to prevent injury. If you become injured, you can't train, you get irritable, and we all suffer.

Your interval-training module can be accomplished in a number of ways: riding a bicycle, using a stationary bike, working out on a stair-climbing machine, running on a treadmill, or jogging around your own backyard (or someone else's for that matter). All you need is a pair of running or cross-training shoes, your exercise machine of choice (if required), your body, and a timepiece with a second hand. Work out every other day for best results.

If you have never trained before, start from day 1. But if you have been participating in a consistent aerobics program and can endure at least 15 minutes at a comfortable "huffing and puffing" steady state, then move on to section II. Sections II and III teach you a variety of intervals. If you have already had at least a year of experience with interval training, try section IV, pyramids. Section V includes speed bursts and speed play. These are fun alternatives to spice up your cardio interval program.

# SECTION I: DEVELOPING AN AEROBIC BASE

For the first month, your goal is to gradually increase the duration of your effort interval (sustained activity) to develop an aerobic base. This increase should be almost imperceptible—similar to a crab sitting in a tub of water that's beginning to boil (or for vegetarians, similar to the slow steaming of some organic Swiss chard). Work out every other day.

• Day 1. Warm up for five minutes with some easy pedaling, climbing, or walking. When you feel ready, pick up the pace to a speed at which you can carry on a conversation but are beginning to huff and puff. Hold this pace for a comfortable five minutes. Recover with a five-minute active rest of easy pedaling, climbing, or walking. Take a few minutes to stretch, and you're done for the day.

• Day 2. Warm up for five minutes with some easy pedaling, climbing, or walking. If you are sore from your previous workout, turn this into a recovery day by continuing a warm-up pace for another seven minutes. If you feel ready for a challenge, pick up the pace to a speed at which you can carry on a conversation but are beginning to huff and puff. Hold this pace for a comfortable seven minutes. Then recover with a five-minute active rest of easy pedaling, climbing, or walking. Take a few minutes to stretch, and you're done for the day.

## Check Your Form

Always pay attention to your form during your effort interval and recovery interval. Are your knees tracking over your toes, not beyond? Is your head up? Is your spine extended? Are your shoulders and arms functioning with resilient strength? Hopefully the answer is yes to all of these. If not, become more aware of your body next time, or turn to "Torture and Punishment: The Dark Chapter."

• Day 3. Warm up for five minutes with some easy pedaling, climbing, or walking. When you feel ready, pick up the pace to a speed at which you can carry on a conversation but are beginning to huff and puff. Hold this pace for a comfortable nine minutes. If you feel light-headed, dizzy, or extremely short of breath at any time during your nine-minute effort interval, take a walking break. Recover with a five-minute active rest of easy pedaling, climbing, or walking. Take a few moments to stretch, and you're done for the day.

• Day 4. Warm up for five minutes with some easy pedaling, climbing, or walking. When you feel ready, pick up the pace to a speed at which you can carry on a conversation but are beginning to huff and puff. Hold this pace for a comfortable 11 minutes. If you begin to feel uncomfortable at this vigorous pace, slow down. Recover with a five-minute active rest of easy pedaling, climbing, or walking. Take a few moments to stretch, and you're done for the day.

• Day 5. Warm up for five minutes with some easy pedaling, climbing, or walking. When you feel ready, pick up the pace to a speed at which you can carry on a conversation but are beginning to huff and puff. Hold this pace for a comfortable 13 minutes. If at any time you feel uncomfortable, slow down. Recover with a five-minute active rest of easy pedaling, climbing, or walking. Take a few moments to stretch, and you're done for the day.

• Day 6. Warm up for five minutes with some easy pedaling, climbing, or walking. When you feel ready, pick up the pace to a speed at which you can carry on a conversation but are beginning to huff and puff. Hold this pace for a comfortable 15 minutes. By now you should feel comfortable at this steady state, which should be just below your anaerobic threshold. Recover with a five-minute active rest of easy pedaling, climbing, or walking. Take a few moments to stretch, and you're done for the day.

• Day 7. Warm up for five minutes with some easy pedaling, climbing, or walking. When you feel ready, pick up the pace to a speed at which you can carry on a conversation but are just beginning to huff and puff. Hold this pace for a comfortable 17 minutes. Recover with a five-minute active rest of easy pedaling, climbing, or walking. Take a few moments to stretch, and you're done for the day.

*After a week of workouts, you're already moving comfortably in your aerobic zone for 17 minutes straight. If everything feels great, then you are ready to take your program to the next level. If 17 minutes is still a challenge, continue to train at this level for another seven days before you move to day 8 of the program.*

• Day 8. Warm up for five minutes with some easy pedaling, climbing, or walking. Pick up your pace. This time go a bit faster than the previous two weeks—not so fast that you feel the burn, but fast enough that you feel a tad winded during your effort. Pick up your speed, but drop the duration back to 10 minutes. If at any time you feel joint pain, dizziness, or shortness of breath, just slow down to your earlier training pace of the first week. Recover with a five-minute active rest of easy pedaling, climbing, or walking. Take a few moments to stretch, and you're done for the day.

• Day 9. Warm up for five minutes with some easy pedaling, climbing, or walking. Then continue to exercise at the same increased pace you used on day 8, but add one minute to the duration so that your work interval lasts for 11 minutes. If at any time you feel joint pain, dizziness, or shortness of breath, just slow down to your earlier first-week training pace. Recover with a five-minute active rest of easy pedaling, climbing, or walking. Take a few moments to stretch, and you're done for the day.

• Day 10. Warm up for five minutes with some easy pedaling, climbing, or walking. Then pick up your pace to the level used on days 8 and 9. As this increased pace becomes more tolerable, increase your duration to 12 minutes. This faster, longer duration makes you a better athlete. Training fast, just below your anaerobic threshold, is the best way to train unless your body is ready to push past anaerobic threshold and can tolerate lactate. If at any time you feel joint pain, dizziness, or shortness of breath, just slow down to the warm-up pace you used on day 2. Recover with a five-minute active rest of easy pedaling, climbing, or walking. Take a few moments to stretch, and you're done for the day.

• Day 11. Warm up for five minutes with some easy pedaling, climbing, or walking. Then pick up your pace. Another minute won't seem so bad: 13 minutes is your goal today! Keep up the pace you achieved on day 8 unless you feel joint pain, dizziness, or shortness of breath; if you do, just slow down to your earlier day 2 training pace. Recover with a five-minute active rest of easy pedaling, climbing, or walking. Take a few moments to stretch, and you're done for the day.

• Day 12. Warm up for five minutes with some easy pedaling, climbing, or walking. Then pick up your pace to your day 8 level. You guessed it—14 minutes today. Get psyched. Let's go! Keep up your pace unless you feel joint pain, dizziness, or shortness of breath; if you do, just slow down to your earlier day 2 training pace. Recover with a five-minute active rest of easy pedaling, climbing, or walking. Take a few moments to stretch, and you're done for the day.

• Day 13. Warm up for five minutes with some easy pedaling, climbing, or walking. Then pick up your pace. You're almost there. Today's the day—15 minutes at the incredibly awesome pace you established on day 8. You can do it! The faster you become, the fitter you are. Keep up your pace unless you feel joint pain, dizziness, or shortness of breath; if you do, just slow down to your earlier day 2 training pace. Recover with a five-minute active rest of easy pedaling, climbing, or walking. Take a few moments to stretch, and you're done for the day.

• Day 14. Begin with a five-minute warm-up. By now your body is getting stronger and more fit, and you're ready for a new challenge. We're going to break up your program so that you get to work harder and rest harder. Pick up your pace, but for only 15 seconds: 15 seconds at a pace at which you breathe heavily and, yes, feel the burn. This should be the first time in our program that you have experienced the burn (exhilarating, not painful). When 15 seconds is up, slow your pace to active rest, that is, the same speed you have been using to recover and cool down in your previous workouts. Maintain this recovery period for 45 seconds. When that second hand hits the 12 o'clock position, do another 15-second work interval with 45 seconds of recovery. Continue this cycle until you have accomplished 10 work intervals and 10 recovery intervals (that is, 10 minutes of training). Cool down with five minutes of active rest. Take a few moments to stretch, and you're done for the day.

Congratulations, it's time to celebrate! Champagne? Caviar? A big piece of cheese perhaps? One month has passed, and you are still hanging in there. Many people quit in the first month, but not you. Stay pumped. Your reward will be your progress (and some cheese if you want it).

## SECTION II: GETTING TO THE NEXT LEVEL

You are awesome. And to celebrate, from now on you will work out every third day (for example, Monday, Thursday, Sunday, Wednesday, and so on). Why? Because you are working harder and you need the rest. If you find yourself getting edgy on your days off, try a completely different activity—strength training, for example.

It's time now for full-on intervals. Remember that interval training improves both your aerobic and anaerobic power. That means that your sport performance will skyrocket in all areas, from sprint-type activity (bursts of energy) to endurance activity (such as swimming laps).

• Day 15. Increase your anaerobic and aerobic power with speed work. After your five-minute warm-up, do a 15-second work interval with 45 seconds of recovery. Continue this cycle until you have accomplished 12 work intervals and 12 recovery intervals (or 12 minutes of training). Cool down with five minutes of active rest. Take a few moments to stretch, and you're done for the day.

• Day 16. Here we go again. Get ready to rumble—speed work, here we go! Today it's 14 work intervals and 14 recovery intervals. After your five-minute warm-up, do a 15-second work interval with 45 seconds of recovery. Continue this cycle until you have accomplished 14 work intervals and 14 recovery intervals (or 14 minutes of training). Cool down with five minutes of active rest. Take a few moments to stretch, and you're done for the day.

- Day 17. Today you train for more than 15 minutes. Are you ready? After your five-minute warm-up, do a 15-second work interval with 45 seconds of recovery. Continue this cycle until you have accomplished 16 work intervals and 16 recovery intervals (or 16 minutes of training). Cool down with five minutes of active rest. Take a few moments to stretch, and you're done for the day.

- Day 18. After your five-minute warm-up, do a 15-second work interval with 45 seconds of recovery. Continue this cycle until you have accomplished 18 work intervals and 18 recovery intervals (or 18 minutes of training). Cool down with five minutes of active rest. Take a few moments to stretch, and you're done for the day.

- Day 19. This is it. Don't hold back. Let your emotions flow. Let's do it! After your five-minute warm-up, do a 15-second work interval with 45 seconds of recovery. Continue this cycle until you have accomplished 20 work intervals and 20 recovery intervals (or 20 minutes of training). Cool down with five minutes of active rest. Take a few moments to stretch, and you're done for the day.

## SECTION III: A NEW CHALLENGE

Ready for a change? If not, or if you really enjoyed section II, feel free to repeat the section II workout for another couple of weeks. But if you are ready for a challenge, move on to the workout in this section.

- Day 1. Try to keep up your new, challenging pace. This time, after your five-minute warm-up, increase your effort interval to 20 seconds and decrease your recovery interval to 40 seconds. Continue this cycle until you have accomplished 20 work intervals and 20 recovery intervals (or 20 minutes of training). Cool down with five minutes of active rest. Take a few moments to stretch, and you're done for the day.

- Day 2. After your five-minute warm-up, do a 20-second work interval with only 40 seconds of recovery. Continue this cycle until you have accomplished 22 work intervals and 22 recovery intervals (or 22 minutes of training). Cool down with five minutes of active rest. Take a few moments to stretch, and you're done for the day.

- Day 3. After your five-minute warm-up, do a 20-second work interval with only 40 seconds of recovery. Continue this cycle until you have accomplished 24 work intervals and 24 recovery intervals (or 24 minutes of training). Cool down with five minutes of active rest. Take a few moments to stretch, and you're done for the day.

- Day 4. After your five-minute warm-up, do a 20-second work interval with only 40 seconds of recovery. Continue this cycle until you have accomplished 26 work intervals and 26 recovery intervals (or 26 minutes of training). Cool down with five minutes of active rest. Take a few moments to stretch, and you're done for the day.

• Day 5. After your five-minute warm-up, do a 20-second work interval with only 40 seconds of recovery. Continue this cycle until you have accomplished 28 work intervals and 28 recovery intervals (or 28 minutes of training). Cool down with five minutes of active rest. Take a few moments to stretch, and you're done for the day.

• Day 6. After your five-minute warm-up, do a 20-second work interval with only 40 seconds of recovery. Continue this cycle until you have accomplished 30 work intervals and 30 recovery intervals (or 30 minutes of training). Cool down with five minutes of active rest. Take a few moments to stretch, and you're done for the day.

• Day 7. After your five-minute warm-up, do a 20-second work interval with only 40 seconds of recovery. Continue this cycle until you have accomplished 32 work intervals and 32 recovery intervals (or 32 minutes of training). Cool down with five minutes of active rest. Take a few moments to stretch, and you're done for the day.

## SECTION IV: PYRAMIDS

Congratulations! You are the ultimate athlete! And now you are about to enjoy a new test—pyramids. You may have heard of pyramid training with weights, but now you are going to learn to use pyramids in your intervals. Pyramids are advanced and definitely demanding—so much so that you may dread doing them week after week. Pyramids, like any other high-intensity interval training, should be performed only twice a week to provide your body enough time for recovery. If you find yourself not training optimally with pyramids (or just feeling pukey), then take a few weeks off between each pyramid workout. If you find that you absolutely hate pyramids, don't do them at all. But if you're up for an exhilarating challenge, get ready, get set . . . go for it!

• Day 1. After your five-minute warm-up, perform a fast-paced 15-second effort interval. Recover for 15 seconds. Now do a 30-second effort interval. Recover for 15 seconds. Now do a 45-second effort interval. Recover for 15 seconds. Now do a full-minute effort interval! Recover for 15 seconds. Now come down the pyramid with a 45-second effort interval. Recover for 15 seconds. Step down again to a 30-second effort interval. Recover for 15 seconds. Perform your last interval for 15 seconds. Recover for 15 seconds. You're done! Cool down, stretch, and shower.

• Day 2. After your five-minute warm-up, perform a fast-paced 30-second effort interval. Recover for 30 seconds. Now do a 60-second effort interval. Recover for 30 seconds. Now do a 90-second effort interval. Recover for 30 seconds. Now do a full two-minute effort interval! Recover for 30 seconds. Now come down the pyramid with a 90-second effort interval. Recover for 30 seconds. Step down again to a 60-second effort interval. Recover for 30 seconds. Perform your last interval for 30 seconds. Recover for 30 seconds. You're done! Cool down, stretch, and shower.

## SECTION V: SPEED BURSTS

If you enjoyed pyramids, do them again this week. If not, try 30-second speed bursts. Speed bursts are intervals of 30 seconds of effort and 30 seconds of active recovery. Depending on how you feel, you can adjust the effort and recovery intervals. If 30 seconds of sustained effort is too long, try a 20-second effort interval and a 20-second recovery. If that is still too much, try a 15-second effort interval followed by 15 seconds of recovery. Speed bursts should be done only twice a week.

• Day 1. After your five-minute warm-up, perform a 30-second effort interval. Take a good 30 seconds to recover. Then hit it with 30 seconds all over again. Recover again for 30 seconds. Continue this cycle 10 times, until you have trained for 30 minutes. That's enough. You're through for the day. Now cool down, relax, and stretch.

• Day 2. Today is speed play. Speed play is fun and productive. Design your own interval workout. Begin with a warm-up. Then go by feel. If you feel like moving fast—go! When you're ready to rest, rest. Then when you're ready, pick up the speed. Faster! Then slow down when you are ready. Pick it up again when it feels right. Listen to your body. Don't push too hard. Enjoy it. When 30 minutes are up, you're done. This should be so much fun that the 30 minutes fly by. If not, try watching *Larry King Live;* maybe Suzanne Somers and Richard Simmons will be on, arguing about protein versus carbs.

From now on, it's up to you to make your workouts fun. Change your training program from time to time, introducing pyramids, speed bursts, or speed play. Go with the feeling; your body will respond beautifully.

To maintain your aerobic conditioning, plan to run, step, bike, or swim three to four days per week for 20 to 45 minutes.

# 4

# EATING PLANS:

## Food Choices to Get Ripped

Your abdominal program and cardio workout will keep you halfway fit. The other half is eating. Despite low-fat foods and diet programs, Americans are fatter than ever. Diabetes, heart disease, and cancer are on the rise, due to many factors. Unhealthy adults set unhealthy patterns for kids, patterns that are passed on for generations if not corrected. According to the Centers for Disease Control and Prevention, 13 percent of children aged 6 to 11 are obese (a 2 percent increase since 1994). The number of obese teens aged 12 to 19 increased 3 percentage points, from 11 to 14 percent. To put it into perspective, from 1963 to 1980, there was only a 1 to 2 percent increase depending on the age group.

The CDC claims that sedentary entertainment (television, computers, Internet, and so on) and changes in diet (such as increasingly pervasive fast-food meals) indeed result in obesity. Our translation, albeit harsh: If you sit on your butt and eat sugar and processed, nonorganic "food" all day, you will eventually develop diabetes or an obesity-related condition, and you will pass these unhealthy patterns on to your children.

So get smart. Support organic farmers by buying pesticide-free, unprocessed, organic, hormone-free, real food. It will be a little more expensive at first, but if everyone asserts that they want to eat in this healthy way, the markets will respond and the junk food will disappear. Buying junk food, growth-hormone-enhanced food, and altered, unnatural fruits and vegetables does not help the environment, the world, ourselves, or our kids. You will have a better, richer life and your abs will have a great chance of survival if you rely on a more natural means of sustenance. Plus, we want you to be around to buy our next book. Read on to learn some great eating tips that can change your life.

## EATING THE HEALTHY ABS WAY

What if we told you that you could go off your diet, lose your rumbling stomach, be less irritable, eat more calories, eat six times a day, actually lose body fat, and feel great? You'd think it was another scam diet claim. Well, it isn't. We recommend the simple lifestyle change of eating six small meals a day. Eating this way will help stabilize blood sugar, prevent mood swings and energy lulls throughout the day, and provide increased energy to really burn fat. Skipping meals sends the body into starvation fat-storage mode, and most low-calorie diets do not jump-start metabolism at all.

After three weeks of eating six quality meals each day, you will discover that greasy foods and rich desserts are not to die for. They actually will not be as desirable, and you will soon lose your addictive cravings. You will desire exactly what your body needs.

## Eating Rules and Regulations

- Undereating or undersleeping can cause overtraining.
- Schedule meals in advance.
- Become sensitive to your energy needs.
- Don't skip meals.
- Eat two servings of carbohydrates and one serving of protein at each meal.*
- Eating and training speed your metabolism.
- Consume most of your calories early in the day.
- Eat slowly to avoid overeating.

* Peter Lemon, PhD, recommends 0.77 grams of protein per pound of body weight separated into several small meals per day for anybody who does cardio and weight training.

Researchers at Boston's Tufts University concluded that those who eat meals while watching television eat fewer fruits and vegetables and actually consume more pizza and junk food than those who turn off the television while dining. Focus on your eating, not the television. Eat slowly, and be aware of what you are putting into your mouth. Include a combination of protein—such as chicken breasts, fish, egg whites, tofu, nuts, beans, and lean red meat—and carbohydrates, including fruits, vegetables, grains, and breads.

When you diet, you lose muscle, water, and fat. If you cut your calories to less than your metabolism needs to support your muscle, 4 to 6 of every 10 pounds you lose will be muscle. Each time you go on a deprivation diet, your body finds it easier to conserve fat because it actually thinks you are starving.

Skipping calories usually means skipping breakfast. If you miss breakfast, your body will definitely fall into starvation mode, holding on to fat. When you finally eat, you may eat too fast or too much, causing an increase in your fat storage.

Eating frequently and slowly is an effective eating plan for an ultradistance cyclist, a bodybuilder, and you. Be sure one of your meals is after your workout. Your muscles can store about twice as many grams of carbohydrates twice as fast if you consume them within 30 minutes of your workout. This window of opportunity is the best time to replenish muscle and liver glycogen stores for your next workout. When you increase your training intensity, add calories to each meal.

## The All-at-Once Meal

Years ago, to save money because I'm cheap, I tried eating one all-you-can-eat meal each day. My metabolism slowed down, and I actually gained body fat. Furthermore, I became lethargic, and my workouts suffered. I realized my body was efficiently storing fat because I was undereating. At the time, there was no way I would have believed that eating six meals a day would help to increase muscle and reduce fat. Today, I am still cheap, but I eat six meals a day and boast 5 percent body fat.—Tom Seabourne

# EATING LOW FAT

Your newly found abdominal muscles (all muscles, for that matter) need calories to move and grow. Muscles prefer to burn carbohydrates for energy and to use protein for growth and repair. Consuming starchy carbohydrates increases your metabolic furnace, but too much fat is simply stored. At first, fat enhances palatability; most people would choose a calorically equivalent piece of apple pie rather than an apple. After three weeks of correct eating, your "fat tooth" may disappear.

Ten years ago, it was difficult to eat low fat. Now there is fat-free everything. But be careful. Low fat is not always low calorie, and with modern chemicals, preservatives, and processing altering the food itself to reduce fat, there is often no way to tell just what you are putting into your mouth and whether it is really good for you. Try not to avoid food with natural fats and oils, like olives, avocados, and nuts. Don't make these your staples, but include them in moderation. Your body really needs a natural level of fat intake. Too much fat avoidance causes fat storage and a confused metabolism. Be aware that when fat decreases in an off-the-shelf product, sugar is likely to increase. Read the label. If it is fat-free, but the first three ingredients are sugar, corn syrup, and fructose, you are about to bite into a significant number of calories and a significant mood-altering, energy-swinging experience that will eventually work against you. Following are some fat-replacement strategies to help you avoid fat overdose, experience more energy, and, over time, show off your abs:

- Saute in defatted chicken broth instead of oil.
- Substitute a quarter cup (59 milliliters) of applesauce for a like amount of oil in muffin, cake, or cookie recipes.
- Make mashed potatoes with skim milk, soy milk, and powdered butter.

- Use powdered butter or a plant-based butter substitute on steamed vegetables.
- Use fat-free imitation sour cream instead of regular sour cream.
- Use evaporated skim milk instead of butter.
- Use skim milk or soy, rice, or almond milk instead of whole milk.
- Use corn syrup instead of oil in cookie recipes.
- Consume yolk-free egg noodles instead of regular pasta.
- Choose angel food cake instead of high-fat desserts.
- Use nonfat plain yogurt instead of oil.
- Use a nonstick skillet instead of a regular greased pan.
- Use two egg whites instead of one whole egg.
- Replace regular cheese with fat-free or soy cheese.

Initially, it may be difficult fitting meals between breakfast and lunch and between lunch and dinner. Eventually, you will need a mere five minutes to scarf down precut vegetables and chicken or some nonfat yogurt. Keep healthy convenience foods, such as organic carrots or almonds, in your car or desk to snack on. Eat a variety of different protein combinations, complex carbohydrates, and a small amount of monounsaturated and unsaturated fats. Be creative. Fuel your muscles while starving the fat.

# WATER

Approximately 70 percent of your body is water. Water is needed for your body to digest and absorb food, transport nutrients, build and rebuild cells, remove waste products, and enhance circulation. Eight glasses of water are enough for a sedentary couch potato, but not for you. Many people who work out are chronically dehydrated. You need about one milliliter

## Scott's Power Smoothie

Put two to three scoops of a soy or nut-based ice cream in a blender. Add about 6 to 8 ounces (177 to 237 milliliters) of soy milk, an ounce (30 milliliters) of apple juice, half a banana, a tablespoon (15 milliliters) of organic peanut butter, and some soy protein powder if desired (nix the soy protein if you don't need the calories); blend it up, and voila! It is animal-free and dairy-free and tastes great.

of water per calorie expended. That means that if you burn 2,000 calories a day, you will need an additional two liters (about two quarts, or eight cups). If you drink enough water to support your workout, the blood-sludging effects of dehydration will be transformed into super-hydrated peak performance.

Your thirst mechanism may malfunction during your workout. Prime the pump by forcing yourself to sip fluids while training. Contrary to the opinion of some health fanatics, it is not mandatory to drink pure water all the time. Juices are 95 percent water, and oranges 90 percent. Also, soups, grapes, and yogurt are mostly water. Coffee and tea are 99 percent water, but the caffeine produces a moderate diuretic effect. Sodas should really be off limits, as they have virtually no nutritional value at all. Both the sugared ones and the diet ones are just processed, highly marketed goop. Stay away from concentrated juices if possible because most contain high-fructose corn syrup. Read product labels. Just because a product claims to be "all natural" does not mean it is.

# EXERCISES

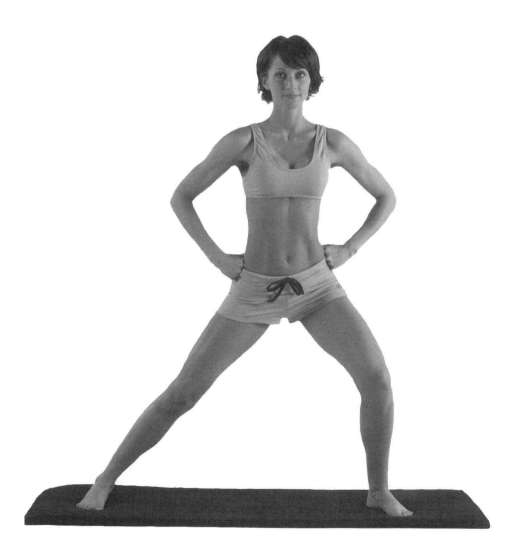

# part II

# TOTAL TORSO:
## Work the Core

The torso exercises in this chapter create awareness of how each core component plays a unique and vital role in the movement of your torso. By understanding basic anatomy and physiology and learning to train your abdominal muscles (rectus abdominis, external and internal obliques, and transversus abdominis) individually, you can then understand the beauty of full-body core training, which we outline in the rest of the book. Remember, achieving athletic abs requires more than just component core training. Like an artist viewing all aspects of her subject, you can be aware of all angles of core training.

## Stimulating Muscles

High-repetition ab training can enhance muscular endurance. The first improvements are due to neurological efficiency as you learn to recruit muscle fibers in your abdomen. Further improvements come from strengthened connective tissue. Stronger tendons and ligaments support your newfound abdominal strength.

Ab training increases the size of the contractile proteins within your abdominal muscle fibers. Each muscle fiber is like an elongated cylinder that generally extends the length of the muscle. Beneath the cell membrane are numerous threadlike structures that contain the contractile proteins of muscle. The thicker, darker filaments are made of myosin, and the thinner, lighter filaments are made of actin. Actin and myosin grow during your rest between workouts, which increases the size and cross-sectional area of the abdominal muscle fiber.

A motor neuron transmits an electrical charge to an abdominal muscle via a network of mainly sodium ions outside the neuron and predominantly potassium ions inside the nerve. The inside of the cell has a less positive charge than the outside of the cell.

The axon that carries the impulse is blanketed with a lipid (fat) cover called a myelin sheath. One function of the myelin sheath is to insulate impulses traveling along the same neuron since neurons are made up of many nerve fibers.

Your muscles need glycogen, ATP, and innervation to become active. Glycogen is the storage form of sugar in muscles. Glycogen is broken down into ATP. In order to contract, muscles require ATP. A stimulus to a motor unit contracts your abdominal muscles on an all-or-none basis; that is, a muscle fiber contracts all the way or not at all. One motor neuron may innervate 1,000 muscle fibers in your obliques to execute a twist, while another motor neuron may activate only 10 muscle fibers to blink your eye.

# Key Points for Torso Exercises

Be sure your body is balanced before you begin.

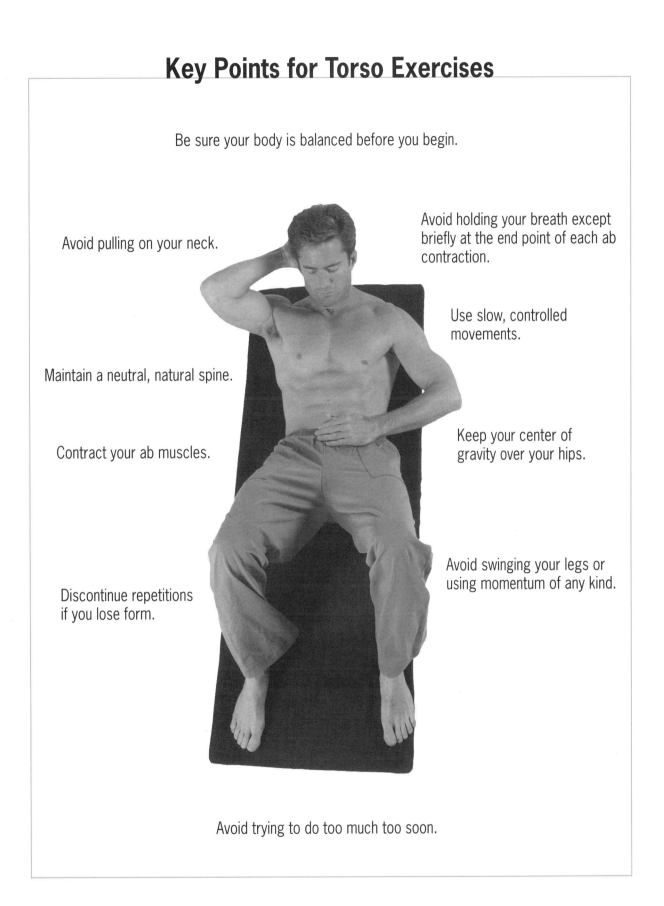

Avoid pulling on your neck.

Avoid holding your breath except briefly at the end point of each ab contraction.

Use slow, controlled movements.

Maintain a neutral, natural spine.

Contract your ab muscles.

Keep your center of gravity over your hips.

Discontinue repetitions if you lose form.

Avoid swinging your legs or using momentum of any kind.

Avoid trying to do too much too soon.

# RECTUS ABDOMINIS

Bruce Lee took advantage of his time by training his incredible abs unnoticed while sitting in boring meetings. He isometrically contracted his abs by pressing his lower back into a chair. There was no apparent movement, but his rectus abdominis muscles were receiving a secret, awesome workout.

Your torso is a vital area for you to tone and strengthen if you want to increase your power. Torso exercises stabilize the spine, protecting you from injury. Abdominal muscles allow your torso to turn, twist, and bend. Your waist connects your upper and lower body to generate the tremendous torque necessary for dynamic punching and kicking. Solid abdominals are essential to make this connection. Strong core muscles also enhance your balance, protecting your internal organs.

The set of abdominal muscles referred to as the "6-pack" is the rectus abdominis, and in reality it is a "10-pack"—go ahead, count them. This muscle group originates on the pubic bone. The insertion (end of the muscle that is attached to the body part to be moved) is on the cartilage of ribs 5 through 7 and the xiphoid process (the lower tip of the breastbone). The rectus abdominis is a straplike muscle designed for smooth, long movement. Its main purpose is to raise your body from bed each morning. The simple crunch trains this muscle group by flexing the trunk forward.

For perfect crunches, begin each repetition as if you were in slow motion. Contract your rectus abdominis, exhaling as you let your muscles pull your shoulder blades up off the floor. Exhaling on each repetition allows you to squeeze your abs without arching your back. Inhale on the return to prepare you for the next contraction; expand into the neutral spine position without relaxing fully, keeping the abs active.

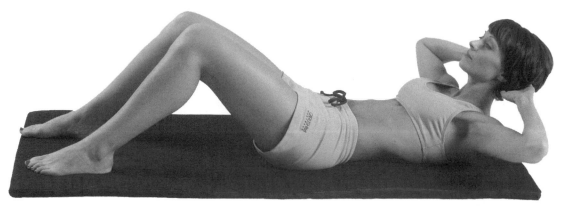

Firming your abs requires good technique and commitment to training, not expensive equipment. For the perfect crunch, curl your head and shoulders a few inches off the floor, focusing on your rectus abdominis and using your abs to lift your shoulders off the floor.

Beware of infomercial abdominal machines. Many of these products make false claims, use only a one-dimensial approach to ab training, are cheaply made, and are not really properly aligned, tested, or designed for safe, repeated use. To firm up your abs free of charge (well, we hope you paid for the book), lie on your back with your knees bent, your chin resting forward toward your chest. Curl your head and shoulders off the floor (without momentum or the use of a crane) upward and forward until your shoulder blades leave the floor. Follow this progression: Tilt, curl, flex for two seconds, then uncurl, untilt. Focus on flexing your rectus abdominis. The range of motion is only a few inches. It should feel as if you are working your upper abs more because the top of your rectus abdominis is thinner than the layer toward the pubis. Perform 10 repetitions. Use your rectus abdominis muscles to raise your body, not your head and neck. If crunches are too difficult, raise yourself off the floor with your arms and perform just the down phase of the crunch.

You can modify your arm position to change the degree of difficulty of crunches. The least resistance occurs when your arms are straight and outstretched along the sides of your body. Level 2 of difficulty is to cross your arms over your chest. Level 3 is elbows bent, fingertips to your ears, or arms extended up; either arm variation adds more resistance to the crunch.

To perform a reverse crunch, lie on your back with your knees flexed to your chest. Place your hands under your hips. Keep your knees together as you bring your feet toward the floor without touching it. Hold for three seconds, then slowly draw your knees back to your chest. It should feel as if you are working the lower part of your rectus abdominis because your hip flexor muscles (iliopsoas) are assisting.

When you attempt to train your abs, the hip flexors (iliopsoas), which are more powerful muscles, do most of the work. This is the main reason that, when done incorrectly, crunches (or anything for that matter) can be a disappointing waste of time. Even when you perform a crunch correctly, your rectus abdominis begins the movement but your hip flexors cannot help but become involved, especially if you attempt to perform crunches quickly with nonmuscular momentum. By raising the torso slowly and coming up only part of the way (full sit-ups have been known to be a big no-no for some time now), you can target your rectus abdominis instead of your hip flexors.

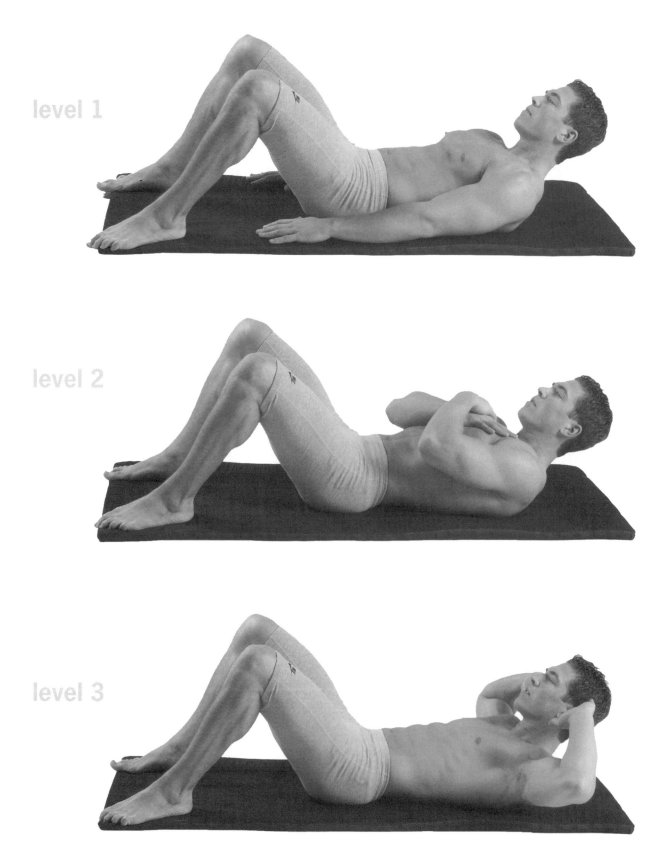

Modify your arm position to increase the difficulty: (a) level 1, arms straight at the sides; (b) level 2, arms crossed over the chest; (c) level 3, elbows bent, with fingertips at ears.

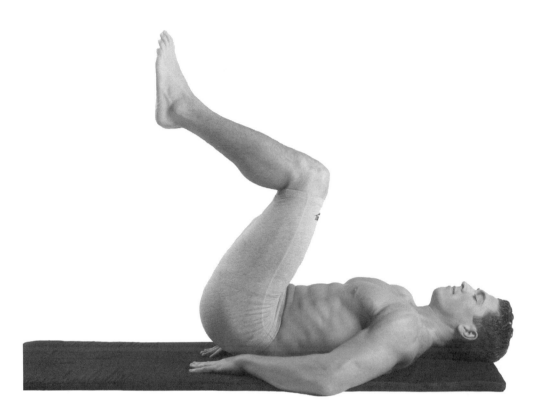

For the reverse crunch, start with your knees near your chest, then lower your feet toward the floor. This move involves your hip flexors to help your abs.

If you anchor your feet under a sofa, table, or gym bar or have a partner hold your feet, you work mostly the hip flexors because you naturally pull against the anchor with your legs. This diminishes the role of the abs in the activity. With your feet anchored, your back may arch, which strains the quadratus lumborum (lower-back muscles).

## OBLIQUES

When you are wearing boots and being somewhat lazy taking them off, you use the toe of one boot to push the heel of the other boot to remove it, and then use your real toes to remove the other boot. You use your obliques in this example of straight and twisting movement. You would probably use them in some capacity as well if you bent over or twisted to pull your boots off with your hands.

Your internal and external obliques cause your trunk to flex as well as to rotate when they contract one side at a time. But when both sides contract simultaneously, your trunk flexes forward. Oblique twists work well to train these muscles.

For the oblique twist, curl your trunk up and diagonally so that your left armpit moves toward your right hip or your right armpit moves toward your left hip. Avoid twisting your elbow toward your knee at the top of your crunch. Instead, raise your elbow toward your opposite knee at the beginning of each repetition in a slow, twisting arc.

Your obliques are used in almost every activity, so train them well. Side bends train your quadratus lumborum, not your obliques, because the torso is not twisting. It is bending to the right and left, which is a different action. The twisting of the torso is the key to training obliques.

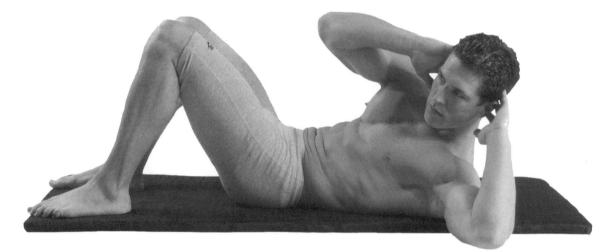

For the oblique twist, curl your arm toward the opposite hip. The key to toning obliques is in the twisting of the torso. Lift your elbow toward the opposite knee in a slow arc.

## External Obliques

A right cross or a left hook is initiated with a twisting action of your powerful obliques. Your external obliques are the "hands in your front pocket," fingerlike muscles that angle inward like the base of a pyramid. Their origin is on ribs 5 through 12, and their insertion is on the iliac crest (top of the hipbone) and pubic bone. Your obliques are thin muscles. They are not designed for heavy resistance training. They wrap around the torso, enclosing the internal structures. The obliques act as a suit of armor to protect and support. These are the muscles you notice when you lift a heavy object. They protect your abdominal area during straining, sneezing, forced expiration, or bearing down. Strong obliques help to pull, lift, or push heavy objects. They steady the torso to keep gravity from pulling you out of a neutral position while standing or sitting. Your obliques help you to balance and move your pelvis and lower back. You activate these muscles on both sides by bending your trunk forward and on one side by bending sideways with rotation. To train your obliques, follow the same technique as the crunch, except raise your upper body at an angle to the right or to the left.

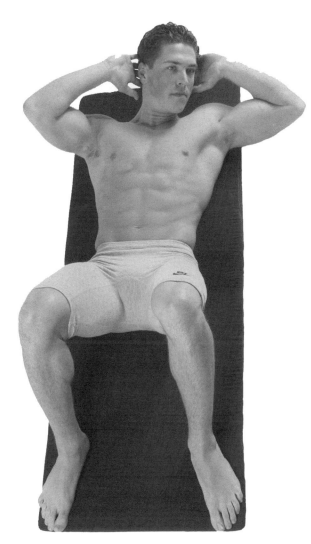

To train the external obliques, follow the directions for the crunch, except angle your upper body to the right or left when you lift your shoulders off the floor.

## Internal Obliques

Imagine that you are facing someone who for no reason at all throws a punch at your face. Being the athlete that you are, you deftly tilt your body sideways out of harm's way. Your internal obliques saved your face. Your internal obliques are under your external obliques and surround your waist. Think of these as the "hands in your back pocket" muscles, fingerlike muscles that resemble the top of a pyramid. They are shaped like an inverted V. Internal obliques stabilize your trunk. Your obliques are the only abdominal muscles constantly active during standing. They function while you are in an upright posture to brace your torso. The origin of the internal obliques is the iliac crest. They insert on ribs 9 through 12. It's best to train the internal and external obliques simultaneously.

# TRANSVERSUS ABDOMINIS

In ancient times, it was said that a master martial artist could exhale through pursed lips with such force that he could kill an unsuspecting fly. This is legend, of course, but such forceful exhalations are one way you can train your transversus abdominis.

The transversus abdominis is another set of stabilizer muscles in your abdomen. They run horizontally. The origin of these muscles is the cartilage of the last six vertebrae, the iliac crest, and the lumbar fascia (a sheet of connective tissue that covers muscles in the lower back). The insertion is the xiphoid process and pubic bone. Their primary purpose is to enable you to force an expiration, such as a cough or sneeze. Simply exhaling through pursed lips stimulates your transversus abdominis.

# 6

# CORE EXERCISES:

## Six-Pack Attack

Core training is important for preventing sport-related injuries. For example, striking a forehand or backhand in tennis begins from the core. A player with an underdeveloped core may suffer one chronic injury after another. Core training could be the key to preventing back pain, strains, and other nagging injuries.

Begin with basic (but clever) trunk stabilization movements. Lie on your back and lift your arm and opposite knee while maintaining a neutral spine. Perform this movement with both sides of your body.

Next try pelvic tilts. Lie flat on your back and bend your knees, keeping your feet flat on the floor. Extend your arms out to your sides. Pull your abdominal muscles in as you tilt your pelvis, tightening your buttocks. Flatten the natural arch of your back against the floor. Hold your abdominals flexed for three seconds as you exhale. Then relax and take a deep breath. Do 10 repetitions.

A basic trunk stabilization exercise like this one can increase your core awareness.

The pelvic tilt is a simple exercise that makes you more aware of your abs.

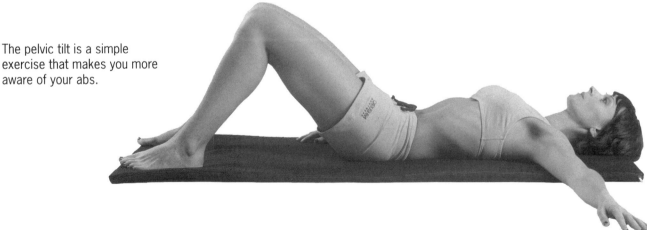

# Key Points to Perfect Ab Work

Perform all exercises in good form.

Contract abs without the use of momentum.

No sloppy movements. Awareness is your weapon.

Pause in the contracted position and relax the contraction.

Be precise in your movement to become more efficient and effective.

Connect mind and body. Focus on the muscle you are working.

Breathe through all moves, lengthening your spine with each breath.

Let grace, speed, and a fluid motion power all movement.

Pull power from the core.

Reach momentary muscular failure in 8 to 12 efficient repetitions.

## Core Strength Test

Good news. If you don't own weights, don't panic. Your body weight is enough to provide resistance for your training. ("Oh, thanks a lot," you may say.) Everyone can use his or her own body weight for resistance training, which is a relief in case you are ever stranded on a desert island and really have to wing your own workout program.

For now, though, get on your knees and place your palms in front of you. If you happen to be on a desert island with our book, good for you. We hope the sand is comfortably warm. Pull your pelvis in, tightening your buttocks. Now, contract your abdomen in as far as it will go. Learn to breathe while your abdomen and buttocks are pulled tight.

The "pull-in" abdominal contraction actually occurs on each exhalation, not by sucking in and holding on each inhalation. You will learn to maintain each position, moving deeper into the contraction, breathing normally throughout. If you have trouble holding your abdomen and gluteals firm, you need to practice. Try this exercise fully with one slow breath, then practice maintaining the ab contraction during two and then three breaths. On the multiple-breath repetitions, maintain the position on breath 1, then contract deeper on breaths 2 and 3.

# CORE TRAINING

Cough! Did you feel your abdominals contract? Cough again and, without relaxing, continue to exhale, hold your contraction for three seconds, and then relax. This is abdominal training as well.

Keep your motion slow and controlled throughout the following exercises. Do not use momentum to complete the exercise. Focus on using your core muscles only; that means keeping your form perfect. We will accept nothing less.

Exercises should be performed in the order given at first. Once you are familiar with the exercises, vary the order to provide a different stimulus to aid your training progress. Simply changing the order of your exercises challenges your muscles into new growth.

Levels 1 through 3 indicate the intensity of exercise variations, from least to most intense. If there is no level designation, you can increase intensity by adding repetitions. Add 10 repetitions to turn a level 1 exercise into a level 2 exercise, and add 10 more repetitions to increase a level 2 exercise to level 3.

Lie on your back. Reach over your head and grab something heavy and solid, such as a chair or partner, for stabilization. Keep your knees slightly bent. Pull your pelvis and legs up so that your knees are above your chest, and then return to the beginning position.

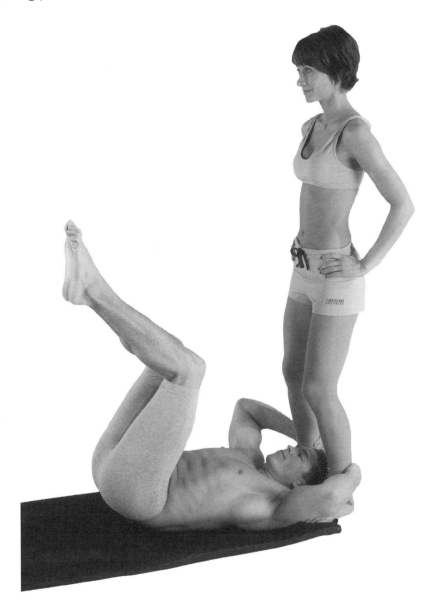

# CRADLE

Lie on your back. Put your fists under your buttocks to form a cradle. Raise your legs 12 inches (30 centimeters) with your knees slightly bent. Raise your head and shoulders slightly off the ground. Then contract your abdominals to raise your legs until your feet are above your pelvis. Thrust your heels toward the ceiling in a short, controlled range of motion while you exhale, contracting your abdominals. Release, returning your feet to a position above your pelvis. After completing your repetitions, lower your legs to the ground.

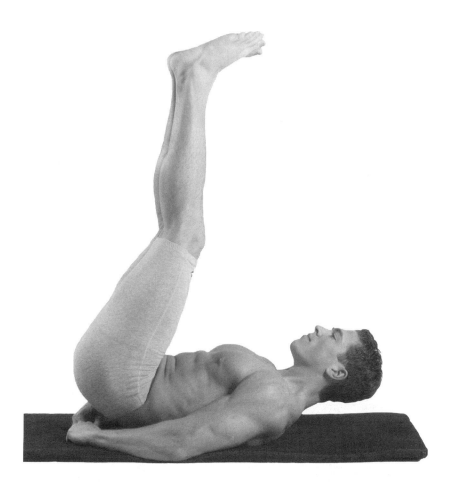

Stand in front of a chin-up bar. Grab the chin-up bar with both hands in a grip a bit wider than your shoulders. Cross your ankles, bringing your knees toward your chest. Pause at the top of the movement for a second and then slowly lower your knees a few inches. Repeat.

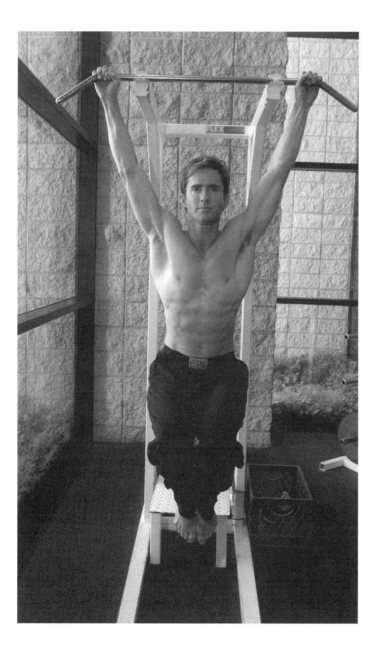

# CURLING CRUNCH VARIATION

Begin in a crunch position with your knees bent 90 degrees and your feet raised. Place your hands by your ears and slowly raise your shoulders off the ground, trying to touch your pelvis to your ribcage. Exhale as you move through this range of motion. Don't let your hips move.

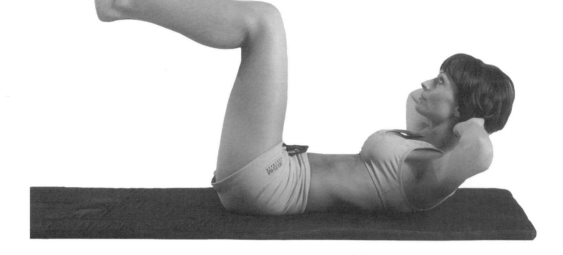

# CURL

Lie on your back with knees bent and comfortably apart and feet on the floor. Use the abdominal muscles to pull the belly in flat. Hold the abdominals flat and curl up as high as you can without letting the lower back come off the floor. The head, neck, and shoulders should curl up as one unit. Hold for a second then slowly lower back to the floor.

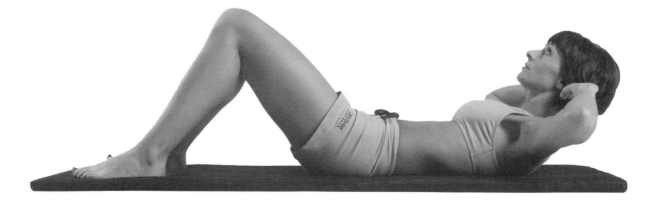

Lie on your left side. Raise yourself up on your left elbow, keeping your elbow at a 90-degree angle with your shoulder, relaxing your neck (a). Contract your abs to keep a tight, straight line from ankles to head. You may balance yourself with your right hand, if you need to (b).

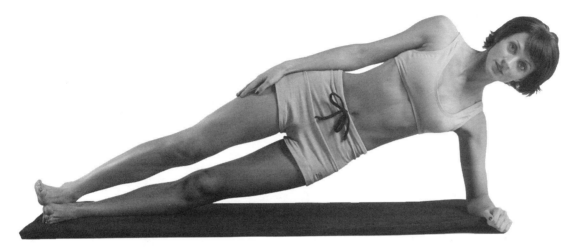

a

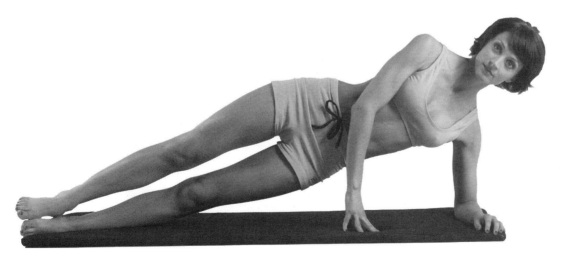

b

# OPPOSITE ARM AND KNEE LIFT

Lie on your back with arms at your sides, knees bent, and feet on the floor. Contract your abdominals, pulling your abdomen in toward the spine. Keeping the abdominal muscles pulled in tight, lift your left foot off the floor. Keep your knee bent until the calf is parallel to the floor. Simultaneously exhale and raise your right arm over your head. Keep your abdominal muscles contracted throughout the movement. Bring both the arm and the leg back to the starting position. Repeat the same movement on the other side.

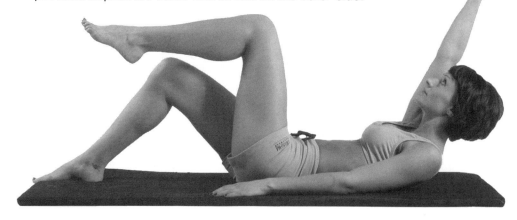

# ISOMETRIC CONTRACTION

Lie on your back with your legs extended above the floor, abdominals contracted as in a curl or crunch position. Raise and lower your arms from your shoulders, as if you were flapping your wings, while focusing on your core muscles. Begin by performing 10 repetitions. Add two repetitions per week until you can perform 30 consecutive repetitions with perfect form. Your abdominal muscles are isometrically contracting for the entire set.

# PERIODIZATION OF CORE EXERCISES

Core training can be cycled to progressively overload the trained muscles. At first, perform the more traditional, level 1, crunch-type, single-plane exercises in a stable position (supported linear movement) at a slow, steady speed. Work on your weaknesses. If your lower back feels weaker than your abs, perform two back exercises for every abdominal exercise. Work your way next to level 2, multiplanar exercises, which are performed at every conceivable angle. Finally, level 3, ballistic movements are performed in a controlled yet unstable position. This doesn't mean that level 3 is unsafe—it simply means that you create your own stability, which challenges you even more, moving you toward full-body multidimensional core training.

Stick to level 1 until you can do 10 repetitions with perfect form. If there is not a more advanced variation to increase the intensity, increase intensity by adding repetitions. Add 10 repetitions to make a level 1 exercise level 2, and add 10 more repetitions to a level 2 exercise to make it a level 3 program.

## SINGLE-KNEE STRETCH

Lie on your back with both knees bent and your feet flat on the ground. Raise one foot off the floor and bring your knee to your chest. Gently pull your knee toward you with your hands and hold it for a few seconds. Slowly release your knee and return your foot to the floor. Do the other leg. You can repeat this simple stretch two or three times on each side, holding your knee for up to 30 seconds.

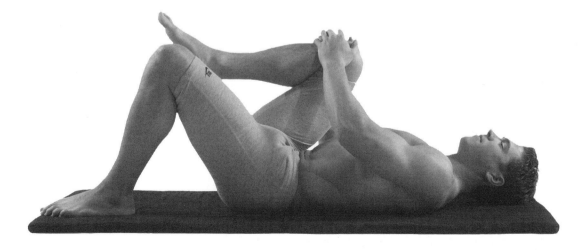

# DOUBLE-KNEE TWISTING STRETCH

Lie on your back with both knees bent and your feet flat on the ground. Spread your arms straight out to the sides with your palms facing up. Keeping your knees bent and your feet together, let both knees drop to the floor on the same side. Don't try to adjust your legs to make one rest perfectly on top of the other; let them fall where they may. Just breathe and try to relax for up to 30 seconds. Gently roll your legs and head back to the center and on to the opposite side. Do this two or three times on each side.

# RELAX AND RECOVER

Lie on your back with both knees bent and feet flat on the floor. Place your arms at your sides with palms facing down. Press the small of your back flat against the mat as you contract your abdominal muscles while exhaling. Hold that contraction for one or two seconds, then relax as you inhale. Repeat 10 or 15 times, then repeat the previous two stretches.

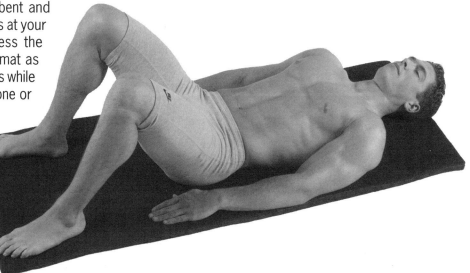

In this lower-ab exercise, notice that the torso is stabilized while the legs move into different positions. Keep your knees soft for each exercise.

Lie on your back, legs straight, keeping your lower back flat on the floor at all times, head flat on the floor as well, and toes turned inward. Hold each level for one minute.

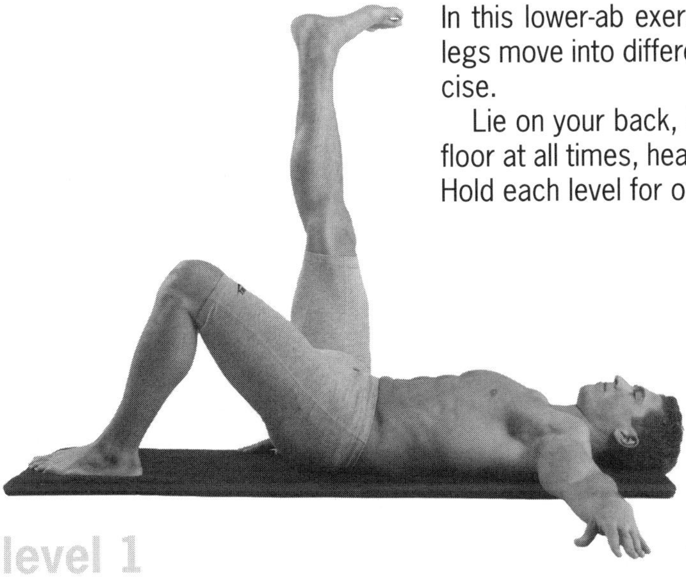

level 1

**Level 1:** Bend one knee, bracing your foot on the floor. Straighten and raise the other leg to 90 degrees, then lower it, taking 3 seconds up and 3 seconds down, with no pause at the bottom.

**Level 2:** Raise both straight legs to 75 degrees and hold for one minute, bending your knees as you begin to fatigue.

**Level 3:** Raise both straight legs to 75 degrees and hold for one minute, keeping your legs straight for the entire minute.

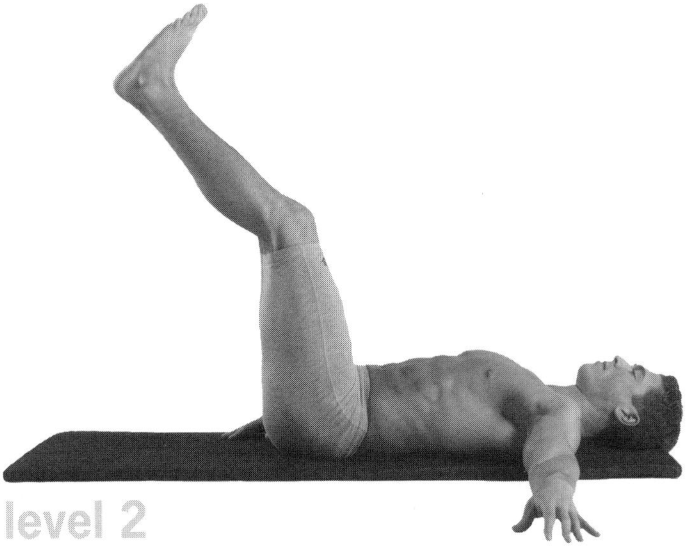

level 2

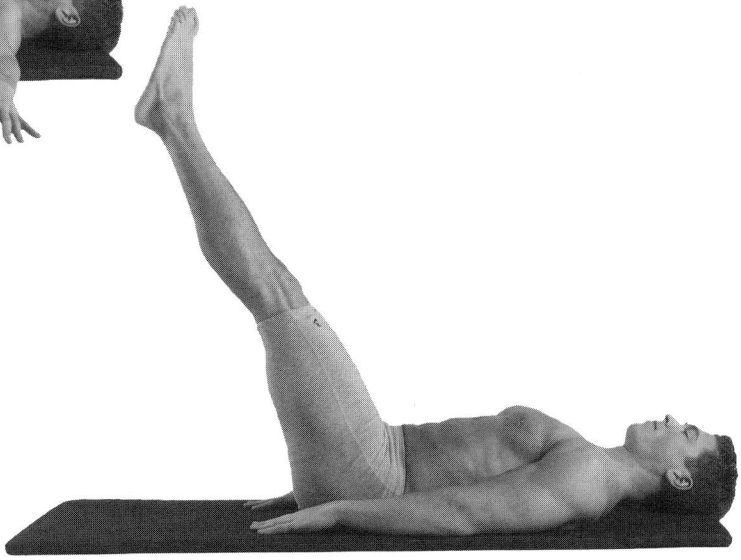

level 3

Notice that the typical rectus abdominis exercises involve a curl-up of the torso, working more of the upper abs. Keep in mind that the rectus abdominis is a long muscle group that can be worked on both ends, which we separate for convenience into *upper* and *lower* abs.

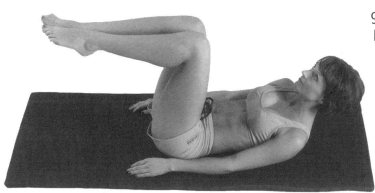

level 1

Lie on your back with your knees and hips bent 90 degrees so that your legs are off the ground, keeping your lower back flat on floor, tongue pressed to the roof of your mouth, and toes pointed in. Curl up for two seconds, one vertebra at a time. Hold for two seconds, then take two seconds to lower. Do not pause at the bottom of the movement.

**Level 1:** Keep your arms on the floor at your hips.

**Level 2:** Cross your hands on your chest.

**Level 3:** Put your hands behind your ears.

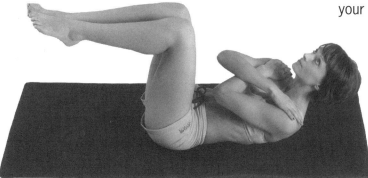

level 2

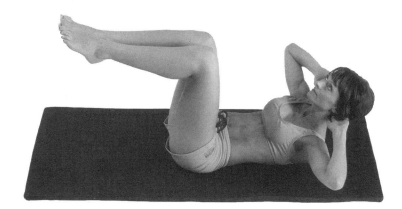

level 3

Lie on your back, your knees and hips bent 90 degrees with your feet off the floor, hands behind the ears. Remember, with your obliques, it is all about the twisting or rotation of the torso. The rotation should be in your trunk, not in your neck. Focus on lifting your shoulder blades off the floor.

**Level 1:** Rise up over two seconds, rotate your torso to the right over two seconds, hold for two seconds, rotate to the left over two seconds, hold again for two seconds, go back to the middle and hold for two seconds, and lower over two seconds. Do not pause at the bottom.

**Level 2:** Follow the same course as for level 1, but rotate your legs in the opposite direction of your upper body. This means that as your upper torso rotates to the right, your knees simultaneously rotate to the left.

**Level 3:** To increase intensity, add 10 repetitions to the level 2 variation.

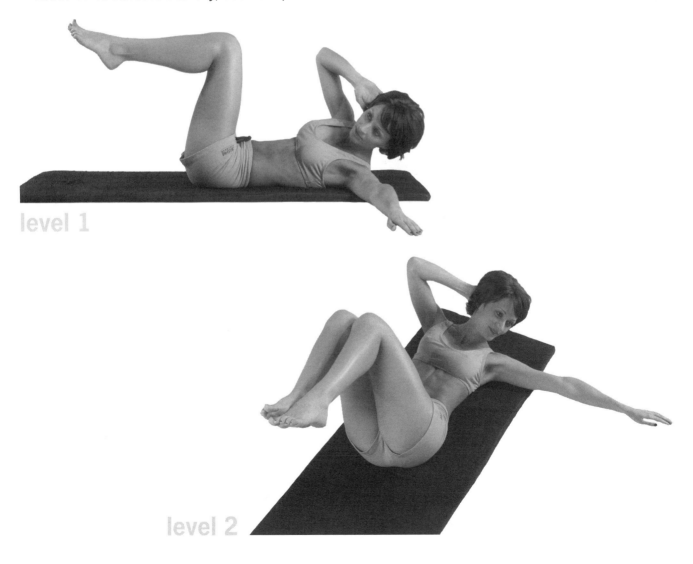

level 1

level 2

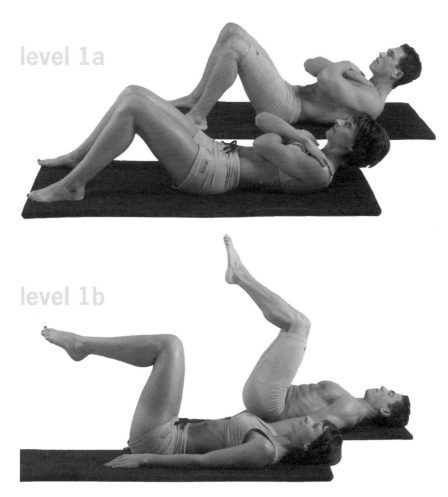

level 1a

level 1b

For level 1, lie on your back with your knees bent and your arms crossed over your chest. Lift your head, neck, shoulders, and shoulder blades simultaneously off the floor in a slow, controlled movement (two counts). Pause for two counts, pushing all remaining air out of your lungs, then slowly lower back to the starting position, barely allowing the shoulders to touch the floor before you begin the next repetition. Keep the abs activated. Exhale as you lift, and inhale as you lower.

Next lift your feet off the floor, with your knees at a 90-degree angle. Pull your abdomen in toward your spine, lifting your hips in two counts until your buttocks and tailbone are off the floor (a reverse curl). Hold for two counts, and then slowly lower yourself. Exhale as you lift, and inhale as you lower.

For level 2, perform both movements together, placing your fists at your temples or extending both arms to add resistance to the slow, concentrated movement. You also can add a weight plate across your chest, just as long as you don't experience neck pain. If neck pain occurs, your form is off and needs correction. You can use a decline bench with your head lower than your feet or with your feet lower than your head for the reverse curl, arms braced behind you or at your sides, to increase intensity.

To increase intensity to level 3, add 10 repetitions to your level 2 exercise.

level 2

Lie on your back with your knees bent, your right hand across your left shoulder, and your left hand beside your left thigh for support. Bring your right shoulder toward your left knee, lifting your head, neck, and shoulder as you bend and rotate at the spine. Keep your hips pressed toward the floor and your abdomen pressed firmly toward the spine. As you begin to rotate, keep traveling upward to get the right shoulder blade off the floor. Pause at the top of the movement, then slowly lower yourself down. Switch sides and repeat the movement. Exhale as you lift; inhale as you lower.

# ABDOMINAL BREATHING FOCUS

Lie on your back with your knees bent, feet flat on the floor, and hands on your abdomen. Take in a full breath, expanding your belly with air. As you exhale, feel the transversus muscle compress your abdomen toward your spine, like squeezing water out of a sponge. Breathe in for four counts, but breathe out for eight counts, making the last four counts of your exhalation a deep abdominal contraction. Finally, try holding the transversus muscle in for a full 60 seconds without holding your breath. Keep breathing normally.

Sit up on your knees, buttocks to heels (rock pose), or sit with your legs crossed, your spine fully extended and neutral. Allow your shoulder blades to pull toward your spine, opening your chest, your chin parallel to the floor. Using a quick, sharp breathing pattern (in yoga this is called "breath of fire"): Inhale fully through the nose, then exhale quickly with short powerful bursts through pursed lips for 30 to 60 seconds. It will make a "shh, shh, shh" sound. Try to perform these breaths from the abdominal region, and let the air come in and out quickly, using forceful contractions from the transversus to exhale.

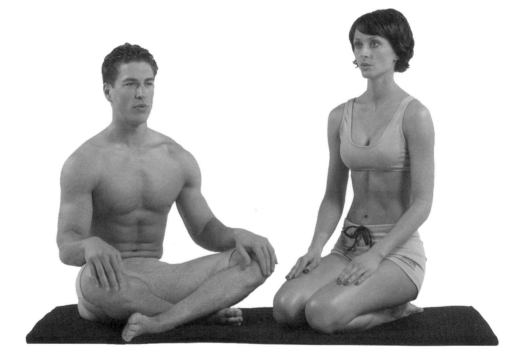

Note: If this exercise makes you dizzy or lightheaded, stop immediately and return to abdominal breathing. Rest for 60 seconds, and then try one more 60-second set.

# Abs Fun Fact

Your abdominals often contract isometrically (without movement) to statically stabilize another movement. Your abdominals also contract dynamically (with movement) to flex your spine. Your hip flexor muscles (at the top front of your legs) are five times stronger than your abdominals. Many so-called abdominal exercises actually employ the hip flexors more than the abs themselves. To help take your hip flexors out of your abdominal workouts, try opening up your knees, placing the soles of your feet together. Another way is press down with the back of your heels on the seat of a chair, hips and knees bent. The contraction of pressing down through the heels opposes the lifting of the legs that engages the hip flexors and often takes away from your ab efficiency.

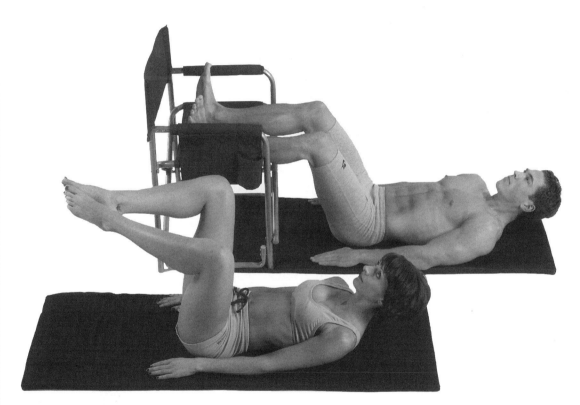

These variations help remove the hip flexors from your abdominal exercises, increasing abdominal efficiency. Put the soles of your feet together or put your heels on the seat of a chair.

# THE SUPER-SLOW WORKOUT

Perform the following exercises in a slow, controlled, rhythmic fashion. Soon you will memorize the order of these moves so that you can slowly move through an entire core routine or kata without stopping between exercises. Allow your body to flow and naturally stabilize itself between moves. This is part of the *Athletic Abs* multidimensional approach.

Begin with a **V sit-up.** Lie on your back with your legs straight. Support your back by propping your elbows behind you. Bring your knees to your chest and then extend your legs slowly until your knees are just slightly bent. Repeat.

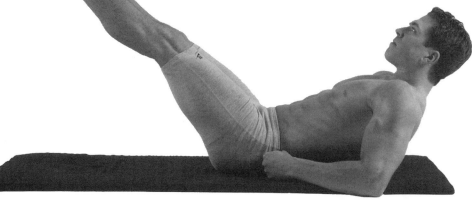

V sit-up

**Flutter kick.** Lie on your back with your legs straight. Support your lower back by placing your elbows on the floor behind you. Lift your legs about six inches (15 centimeters) from the floor. With your knees just slightly bent, alternate lifting each leg as high as possible and very slowly. The opposite leg should remain six inches from the floor. Repeat.

flutter kick

**Leg raise.** Lie on your back with your legs straight. Support your back with your elbows. Raise your feet very slowly and as high as possible. Gently lower them to just six inches (15 centimeters) from the floor. The range of motion is from six inches to as high as possible. Do not use momentum. Keep your knees slightly bent at all times.

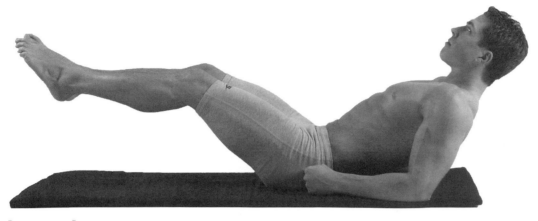

leg raise

**Side to side.** Lie flat on your back with your arms out to your sides. Raise your head and shoulders off the floor. At the same time, lift your feet to a 90-degree angle with your knees slightly bent. Gently allow gravity to pull your legs from one side to the other. Your feet should come no closer than three inches (7.6 centimeters) from the floor.

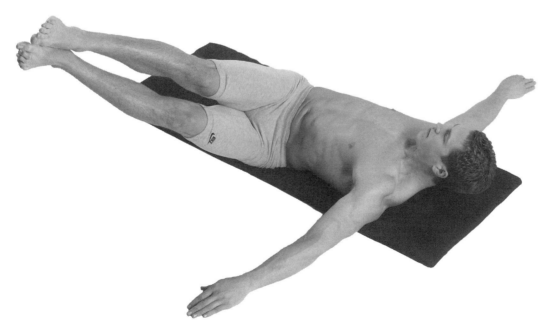

side to side

**Scissors.** Lie on your back. While your elbows support your lower back, extend your legs to the front with your knees slightly bent and raise your feet about six inches (15 centimeters) from the ground. Cross your right leg over your left then your left leg over your right and repeat.

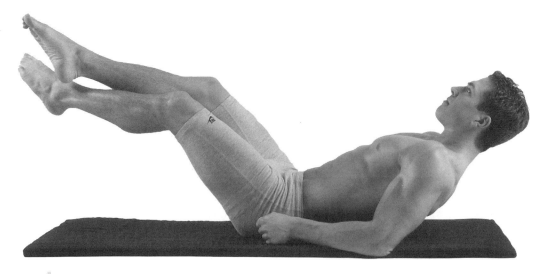

scissors

**Bicycle.** Lie on your back. Use your elbows to support your lower back. Lift your feet about six inches (15 centimeters) off the ground. Extend your right leg by straightening your right knee, and retract your left leg by bending your left knee. Alternate legs, extending and retracting as if you were riding a bicycle with a huge sprocket.

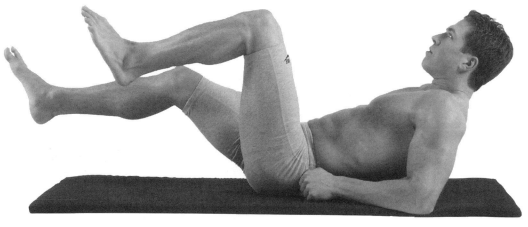

bicycle

**Leg extension.** Lie on your back. Use your elbows to support your back. Bring both knees to your chest and then extend your legs forward and up as high as possible. Keep your knees slightly bent.

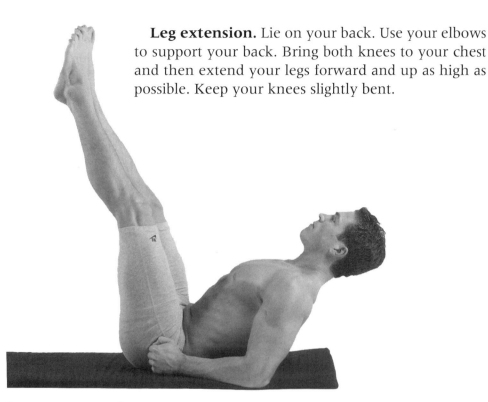

leg extension

**Elbow to opposite knee.** While you lie on your back with your knees bent, interlock your fingers behind your head. Raise your right elbow to your left knee without pulling on your neck with your hands. You should feel the tension in the upper right quadrant of your abdomen (external obliques). Hold for a count of three. Repeat with your left elbow reaching toward your right knee and hold for a count of three.

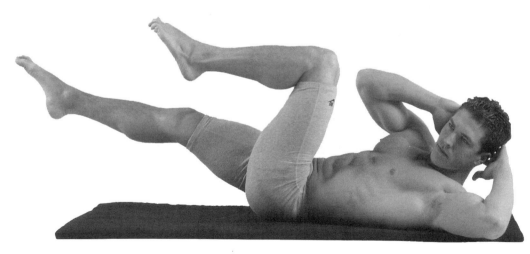

elbow to opposite knee

**Feet up.** Lie on your back. Raise your feet straight up and keep your knees slightly bent. Interlock your fingers behind your head and attempt to bring your elbows up toward the ceiling without pulling with your hands. Simultaneously bring your hips off the floor as you reach your toes toward the ceiling.

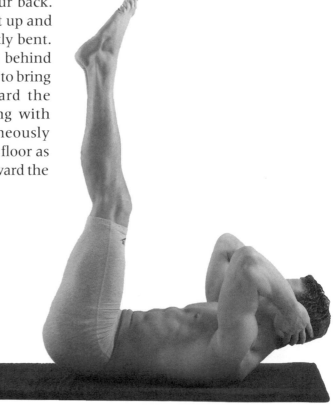

feet up

**Feet out.** Lie on your back. Allow your legs to stretch out to the sides as far as possible with your knees slightly bent. Extend your arms out to the front as you lift your head and shoulders off the floor.

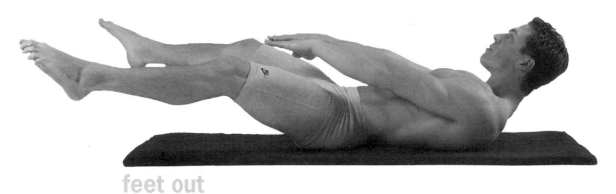

feet out

**Opposite extension.** Lie on your back with your knees up. Interlock your fingers behind your head. Pull your right elbow up to your left knee as you simultaneously extend your right leg out to the front. Hold for three seconds. Bring your left elbow to your right knee and extend your left leg forward. Hold for three seconds.

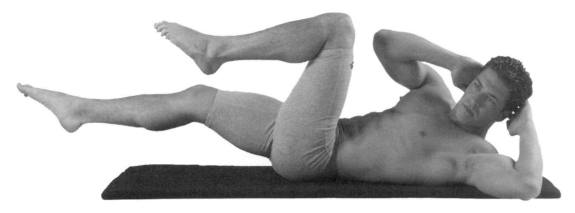

opposite extension

**Leg up.** While lying on your back, prop your left foot up on your right knee. Interlock your fingers behind your head. Raise your right elbow toward your left knee. Hold for three seconds. Release the tension, then repeat. Without changing the position of your legs, raise your left elbow toward your left knee. Hold for three seconds. Repeat. Then switch the position of your legs, so your right foot is propped on your left knee. Repeat the exercise, holding for three seconds.

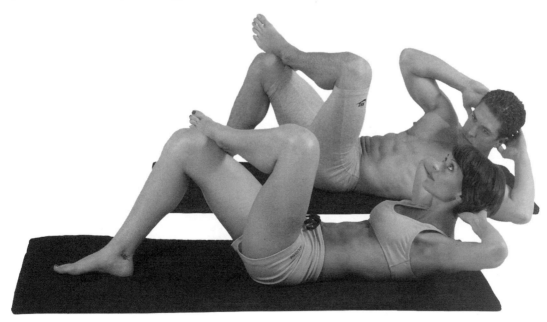

leg up

**Slowly down.** Lie on your side with your feet together and your knees straight. Raise both legs three inches (7.6 centimeters) to the side, and then bring them down slowly.

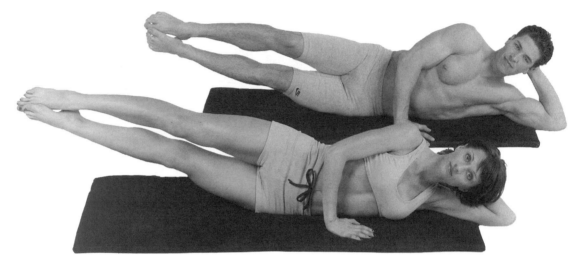

slowly down

**Top leg over.** While lying on your side, cross your top leg over the other leg. Attempt to lift the lower leg three inches (7.6 centimeters) from the floor. Hold for three seconds.

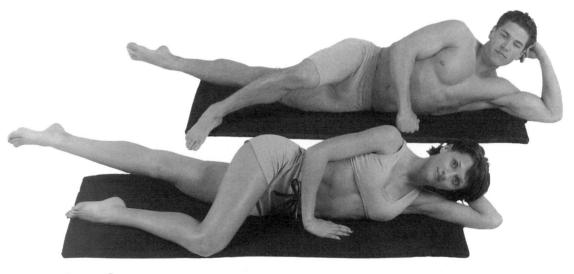

top leg over

**Both feet, same time.** This exercise requires that you hold your legs together and lift them both three inches (7.6 centimeters) off the floor. While lying on your side, gently lift and lower your legs.

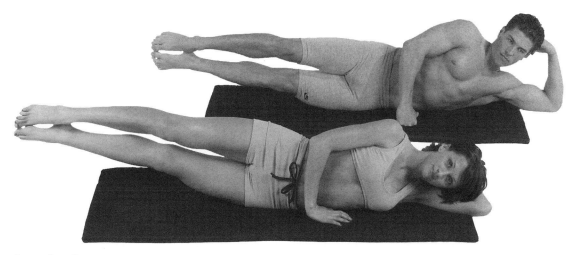

both feet

**Alternate feet.** Lift your top leg one foot (30 centimeters) off the floor. Bring the bottom leg up until it touches the top leg. Then lower the bottom leg to the floor. Finally, bring the top leg down to the bottom leg.

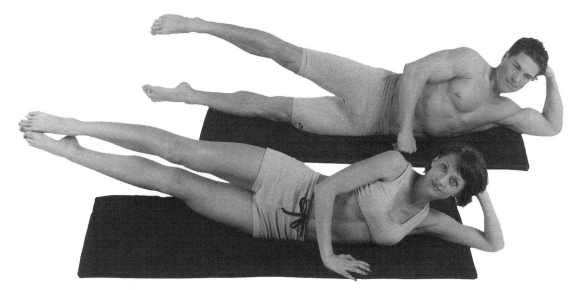

alternate feet

**Side balance.** Put your hands behind your head. Lift your top leg three feet (0.9 meters) off the floor, keeping your feet together and bending your knees. Hold in a static position, contracting your abs to keep your balance. Lower your legs and repeat.

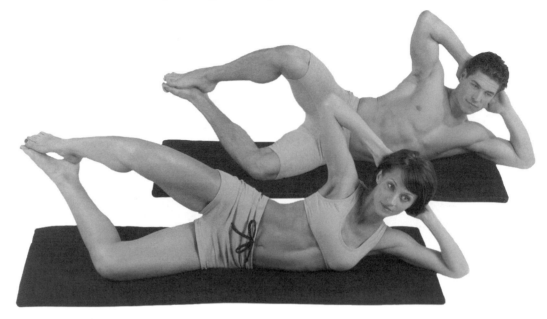

side balance

**Elbow to hip.** As you lie on your side, bring your knees up, keeping your feet together. Interlock your fingers behind your neck. Gently lift your top elbow toward your hip.

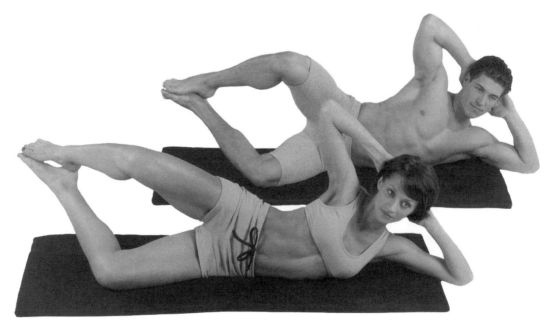

elbow to hip

**Knees up.** Lie on your side, propped on one elbow. Allow your elbow and hip to support your weight. Keep your knees together and hold them as high as possible.

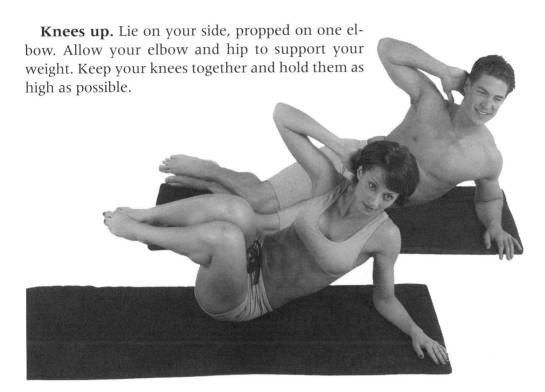

knees up

## THE SUPER ABS ROUTINE

If you are at level 1, perform 10 repetitions for each exercise. To increase intensity, add 10 more repetitions for level 2 and another 10 repetitions for level 3.

**Continuous rotation.** Lie supine with your knees spread and your ankles crossed. Cross your arms over your chest. Perform continuous rotations of your torso, lifting alternate shoulder blades off the floor.

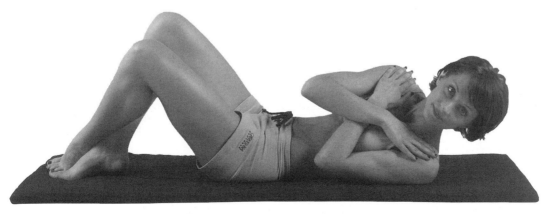

continuous rotation

**Double crunch.** Lift your feet off the floor, knees open, ankles crossed. Perform a double crunch, lifting your shoulder blades and tailbone. Cross your ankles the other way and repeat the continuous rotations and the double crunches.

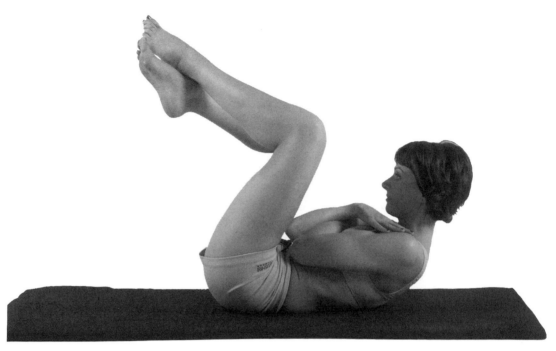

double crunch

**Continuous rotation, arms crossed.** Put your feet down (legs can be straight). Cross your arms over your chest, and do continuous rotations of your torso, lifting one shoulder blade, then the other.

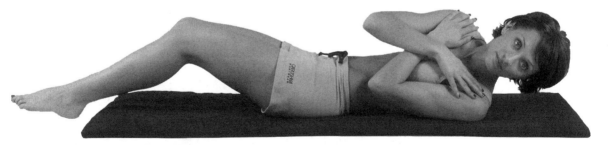

continuous rotation, arms crossed

**Straddle lift.** Lift your legs, keeping them slightly open and soft (pretend you are holding a stability ball between your legs). Lift your hips and your tailbone off the floor.

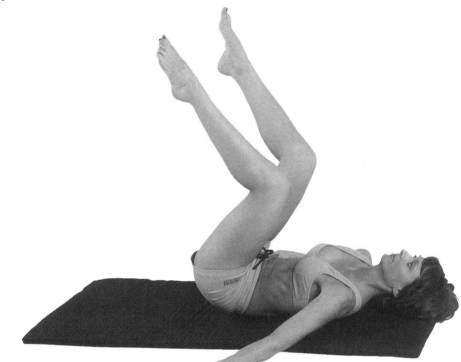

straddle lift

**Oblique crunch.** With your knees bent 90 degrees and ankles crossed, lift your shoulder blades and tailbone and bring the left side of your ribcage toward the side of your left hipbone.

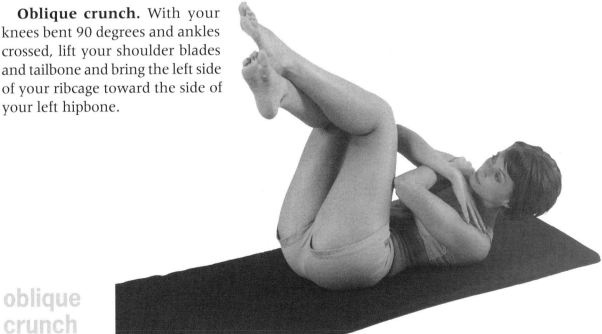

oblique crunch

**Cross.** Finish with long legs, your arms open directly out to the sides. Reach your right arm directly across your chest toward your left hand, fully lifting your right shoulder blade. (Placing your left leg on top of your right leg can help isolate work.) Repeat the oblique crunches and crosses on the left side before returning to the first exercise of the Super Abs routine (the continuous rotations) and repeating the entire sequence on the other side.

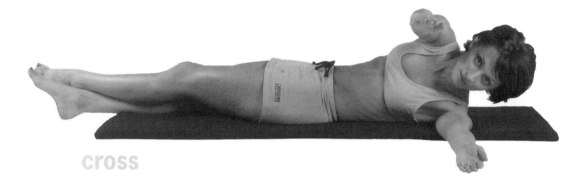

cross

# 7

# BACK STABILIZERS:
## Counterbalance for the Abs

In the old days, there was no such thing as furniture. Humans just sat on their haunches. This is how they ate and how many cultures still use the restroom. Just as a baby can sit for hours playing in a full squat, contemporary Asians are able to squat, waiting for buses on street corners without letting their seats touch the ground.

Asians are more flexible than Americans and statistically have fewer back problems. This is largely due to cultural movement patterns (like in-floor squatting toilets), riding bikes to work, walking between appointments, and leaner bodies due to a better, cleaner diet and higher overall activity levels. Sitting too long in a chair causes stabilizer muscles to atrophy. The fluid-filled disks in the spine succumb to degenerative disease with prolonged sitting. Today, physical therapists use physio balls to re-create the unstable environment that your back needs for optimal health. Sitting on a ball keeps you in constant motion, nourishing your disks and strengthening your spinal erector muscles.

## BALANCING THE ABS AND BACK

It is not beneficial to possess awesome abs with the expense of awesome low-back pain. We have seen people do bizarre exercises in the gym in an attempt to gain awesome abs. One young man placed a 25-pound (11-kilogram) weight on his face while he performed sit-ups. His nose protruded through the hole in the middle of the plate so he could breathe. His new book, *Strange Faceless Abs,* should be in stores soon (we have to get a little wacky).

Performing hundreds of crunches a day may be quite unnecessary and actually harmful to your spinal disks. Crunching forward forces the annulus (ringlike part) of lower-back disks into your spinal nerve, causing pain. After you finish your abdominal workout, it is a good idea to perform some back hyperextensions to move your lower-back disk material back into place, balancing your workout and your abs and back.

### Amazing Agility

I have made over 12 trips to Japan to conduct seminars. I am amazed at the agility of the average Japanese citizen. No kidding—many men and women in their 80s walk briskly, ride bicycles, and squat like kids waiting for buses and trains, putting their bodies in positions that many Americans of the same age would have to call 911 to get out of. I almost had to call 911 when I first used a traditional Japanese floor toilet.—Tom Seabourne

Test the balance of strength between your lower back and abdominal muscles by performing this exercise. Lie on your back, keeping your lower back flat on the floor while you extend your legs toward the ceiling. Slowly drop your legs while attempting to hold your lower back flat on the floor. Your hip flexors eccentrically contract against your abdominals, and your back must resist the downward force of your legs. As soon as your back begins to arch, mark your score.

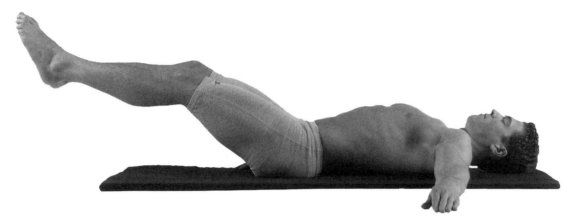

How far can you lower your legs while keeping your lower back flat on the floor? This exercise demonstrates whether your abs are strong enough to counterbalance the pull from your hip flexors.

You may be capable of completing 100 sit-ups in a couple of minutes, but without abdominal strength, stability, and balance, you may not be able to move your legs more than a few inches without your low back curling off the floor. If your legs moved only a few inches (75-degree angle), you display poor abdominal stability. If your legs reached almost all the way to the floor (5-degree angle), your torso strength is excellent.

## PROTECTING BACK HEALTH

When you develop powerful obliques (the abdominal muscles on the sides of your torso), you receive an added bonus of muscular love handles over your hips. Training obliques does not make your waist smaller. In fact, if you overload your muscles, your waist may grow larger because you are increasing your muscle size, but you will look more impressive in a swim-suit. When you contract your obliques, they provide structural support to your spine, like an inner tube being filled.

Sit-ups and crunches do little to equalize the strength in your obliques and back, which are vital for stability. Standing upright, which humans do, requires multidimensional stability. Your abdominal muscles, obliques, and back work together to stabilize your movement, whether you are aware of it or not.

The safest position for the low back is the neutral spine position. Neutral simply means a slight natural curve in the lower back. Our spines are not straight like two-by-fours. Old-fashioned ab training taught a constant contrived adjustment of the spine into an unnatural position. A natural, neutral spine places the least amount of pressure on disks, ligaments, and bones, so we work from that position. Plus, you can absorb impact better in a natural, neutral position than in a forced position that often feels stiff and jarring. The breadth of the natural lordotic curve is individual, like a fingerprint.

Excessive arching and flattening of the back stresses the spinal disks. This can lead to nerve root irritation, degeneration of the vertebrae, and herniated disks. Gravity pulling you out of alignment while you are sitting or standing can cause chronic pain.

Within minutes, gravity and a variety of other factors pull you out of perfect alignment. It takes practice and muscular endurance to stay in a balanced, naturally arched, neutral position. A strong leg base and a slight bend in the knees will help you stay in neutral. Try spending five minutes in neutral. Add two minutes a week until you can sit through your favorite sitcom in neutral.

Practice maintaining a neutral spine while sitting, standing, and exercising. While reading, think about posture. Adjust your spine into pelvic neutrality. Notice how healthy it feels to release unwanted tension. Maintaining a relaxed, buoyant leg base helps provide support, as do opening the inner thighs and including a variety of movements.

To examine your flexibility and balance, lie flat on a hard floor. Where do you feel the heaviest pressure against the floor? Do you feel lopsided, heavier on one side, or are you balanced?

Stand barefoot facing a mirror. Better yet, take all your clothes off to fully view yourself. How is your weight distributed? Are your feet angled in or out? Are your hips even? Are your shoulders level and parallel with your hips? Do your toes and kneecaps face forward? Do you see the sides or back of your hands? Just observe; do not judge. The more you know about your body, the better you can understand your individual needs.

Eighty percent of people will have low-back pain at some time in their lives. Chronic pain in the lower back can be attributed to weak abdominal muscles, tight hamstrings, poor lifting technique, biomechanical abnormalities, or muscle imbalance. Most of these problems can be corrected or prevented through smart exercise and stretching. If you are sitting down, taking pain medication, and expecting your lower-back pain to disappear as you gain weight and become more sedentary, you are in for a rude awakening. The Chinese view pain as blocked energy. Chi, or energy, moves through the body at all times, like steam. Movement creates heat, energy, and blood flow, so the expression "Move it or lose it" has a special significance for lower-back health.

# Key Points for Developing a Strong Back

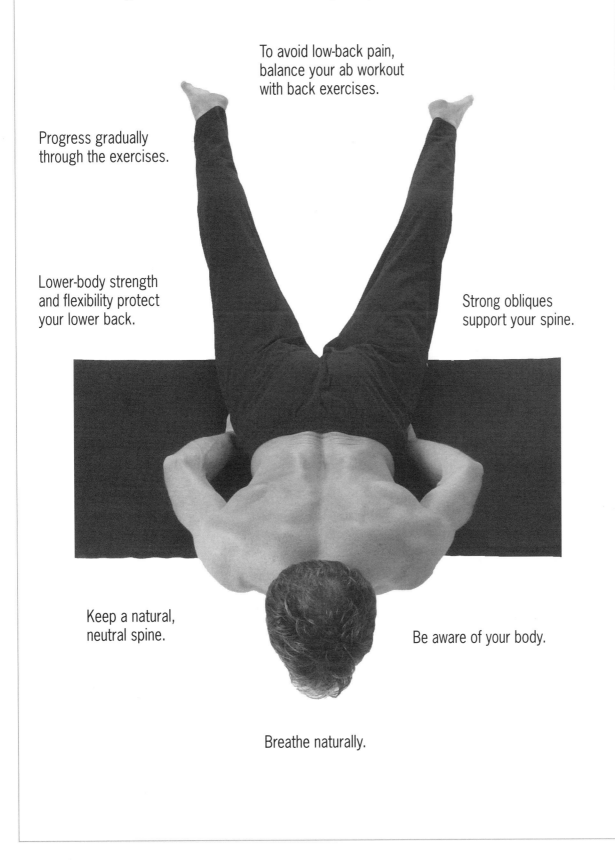

To avoid low-back pain, balance your ab workout with back exercises.

Progress gradually through the exercises.

Lower-body strength and flexibility protect your lower back.

Strong obliques support your spine.

Keep a natural, neutral spine.

Be aware of your body.

Breathe naturally.

# LOWER-BACK EXERCISES

A healthy lower back is a function of lower-body strength and flexibility. Balance between strong abs and a strong back is vital to health, comfort, athletic performance, and injury prevention. The following exercises work primarily the lumbar area of the back but are not limited to only that area. We believe in full-body conditioning. In this case, other muscles of the back are involved as well for a more balanced approach. The erector spinae, quadratus lumborum, and multifidus are the prime movers, but other torso muscles contribute to the synergistic effect of each movement.

People often panic during back exercises because they cannot see exactly what they are doing. It is a great challenge to feel and understand your range of motion and your temporary limits. Be patient. Over time, your back will become stronger and more flexible. Remain conscious of breathing naturally through these exercises. Momentum is definitely an enemy to back training. Proceed gradually through this program, paying particular attention to stiffness or pain in the lower-back area. By moving slowly and efficiently, you can tune in more quickly to your back and its needs. Ease into the forward bend, buttocks to heels, at any time to stretch.

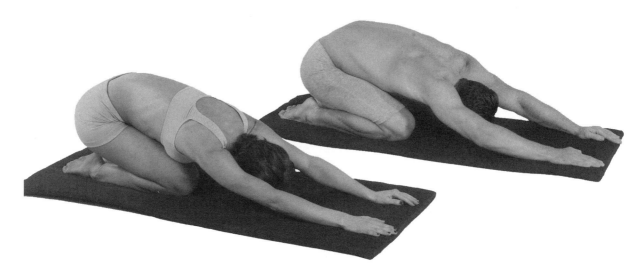

For a good stretch while training your back, ease into a forward bend.

Lie face down on the floor, hands palms up underneath the thighs. Flex your feet with your toes touching the floor. Keep your neck lengthened, face toward the floor. Point each foot, one at a time, and gently arch into an isometrically flexed back position, slowly raising your torso as well. Breathe, relaxing your joints as you strengthen your back. Comfortably keep your shoulders lifted and your upper, middle, and lower back arched. Hold at the top of your range for 10 seconds, breathing as you hold the position. Relax, then repeat two more times.

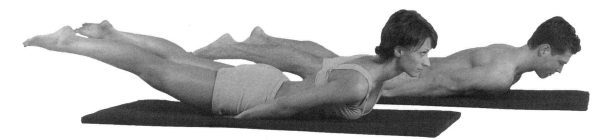

Lie face down on the floor. Stretch your arms over your head, left arm extended, right arm bent with right palm to the floor. Lift your left arm and right leg three inches (7.6 centimeters) off the floor. Keep your leg soft at the knee and your pelvis on the ground. Point and flex your foot if you like, for variety. Repeat with your right arm and left leg, bending your left arm for support. Think "lengthen" as you lift. Do three full sets on each side, holding for 5 to 10 seconds at the top.

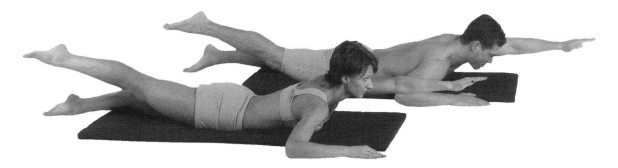

# ALTERNATING BACK LIFTS

Lie face down with a rolled towel placed evenly under your hips. Reach both arms over your head with your legs straight, toes down, feet about hip-width apart. Before moving into the exercise, contract the abdominal muscles and the gluteal muscles to support the lower back. Slowly lift one arm, shoulder, head, and chest as a single unit a few inches off the floor. Pause for a few seconds, and slowly lower to the start position. Be sure to exhale as you lift and inhale as you lower. Repeat on the other side. Alternate sides for five slow sets, holding only briefly at the top.

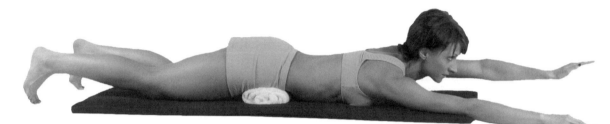

# BENT-OVER SUPPORTED EXTENSION

Standing with your knees bent, bring your torso forward, bracing your hands behind your calves, your elbows bent. You may feel a nice stretch in your legs and back as you ease into starting position. With your hands grasping your legs, extend your back up, allowing your arms to extend fully, hands still braced behind your calves. Exhale on the rise; inhale on the rounded-back return. Repeat five times very slowly, making sure not to keep your head below your waistline for too long. Never perform any "upside-down" exercises right after intense cardio exercise.

# 8

# COMBINATIONS:

## Strengthen the Support Muscles

Establishing a base or foundation is very important for balance, stability, strength, and endurance. Take a building, for example. If it is built on the side of a hill, it needs a certain kind of support. If it is built on marshy land, it needs another kind of support. Your body needs a strong foundation, too. If you are seated with your legs crossed, make sure your "sit bones" (ischial tuberosities . . . sounds like a group of alien spaceships) are your foundation. Sit tall, keeping your lower back neutral, extending your spine, and lengthening through your neck. The abdominals strengthen your support even in a seated position.

You may be used to performing exercises from a seated, stable position. This is somewhat limited, however, like doing only crunches for your core. Crunches are linear and compartmentalized, while overall core conditioning is rotational and multidimensional. The exercises presented here emphasize multidimensional training and force you to train in real-life, full-body situations. After a few months on this program, picking up your child will be easier, and rushing through the airport with a heavy suitcase will not be a problem either (especially after a double iced mocha from Starbucks).

## BEGINNING THE BASE PROGRAM

A strong leg base is vital to greater core strength. As your legs move, so does your core, in a miraculous variety of stabilizing ways.

Stand with your feet shoulder-width apart. Let your arms hang to your sides. Balance your weight evenly on your feet. Contract your thighs by imagining you are drawing your knees upward. This creates a strong, easy base of support.

The pelvis supports the spine perfectly by remaining parallel to the floor in a neutral position. Avoid tucking your tailbone or arching your lower back.

Extend your spine by pressing your feet into the ground. Then stretch your legs upward, starting from the heels to the inner legs to the pelvis. Feel your navel moving in toward your spine and up toward your ribcage. Breathe deeply and evenly as you lengthen upward, relaxing your diaphragm.

Open your chest as your spine lengthens. Relax your shoulders and extend your neck, lifting from the crown of your head. Be sure your chin doesn't jut forward, causing tension. Your neck is an extension of your spine. Feel the length of your spine and remember to breathe. This all sounds complicated and contrived, but it is designed to help you rediscover your natural alignment.

# FOUNDATION-STRENGTHENING EXERCISES

All of the exercises in this chapter strengthen the quadriceps, gluteals, and hamstrings. But because you are training on one leg, the gluteus medius and minimus (the muscles on the sides of the hips) stabilize you. You also use these muscles when you stand, walk, or run.

To further test yourself and understand the core-and-leg relationship, try standing on your right leg while you read the rest of this paragraph. (It is indeed like walking and chewing gum, but we have the utmost confidence in you.) Your right adductor muscles, right internal obliques, left external obliques, right gluteus maximus, left latissimus dorsi, and left quadratus lumborum all contract harmoniously to hold you upright.

Now try standing on your left leg with your right leg raised in various positions to change your body's center of gravity. Then try these with your eyes closed. (Note that you won't be able to read with your eyes closed.) Now experiment by standing with one foot in front of the other on an imaginary line. Then try this with your eyes closed. Lunge forward with eyes open and then closed. Lunge backward with eyes open and then closed. Lunge sideways with eyes open. Try this with your eyes closed. Hop on one leg. Can you close your eyes and do this? Switch legs. Cool, you are awesome and hopefully now more aware of your grounded, strong leg base.

The gluteus maximus is the strongest hip extensor (a muscle that pulls the leg backward). The hamstrings work together with the gluteus when you sprint, climb, or rise from a squat position. In fact, a parallel squat is a great way to train the gluteus maximus.

A diagonal lunge trains primarily the quadriceps muscle. A lunge can also train the gluteus if you keep the front tibia (shin) perpendicular to the floor as the back knee approaches the floor. Press from your heels in your squats and lunges to feel more activation of the gluteus. The gluteals stabilize the pelvis to keep you safe as you continue our program.

Everyone can stand to develop his or her stability muscles for optimal gains in size and symmetry. Leg strength and stability contribute to speed, power, balance, and agility. Traditional bodybuilding programs typically overlook single-leg exercises. Single-limb training is important for developing stability, size, and strength. The following exercises fully prepare your muscles to grow from the inside out.

At first, do 10 repetitions of each exercise. Add 2 repetitions each week until you can perform 20 consecutive repetitions. Level 3 trainees should pause at the bottom of each repetition for a split second.

# Key Points for Building a Firm Foundation

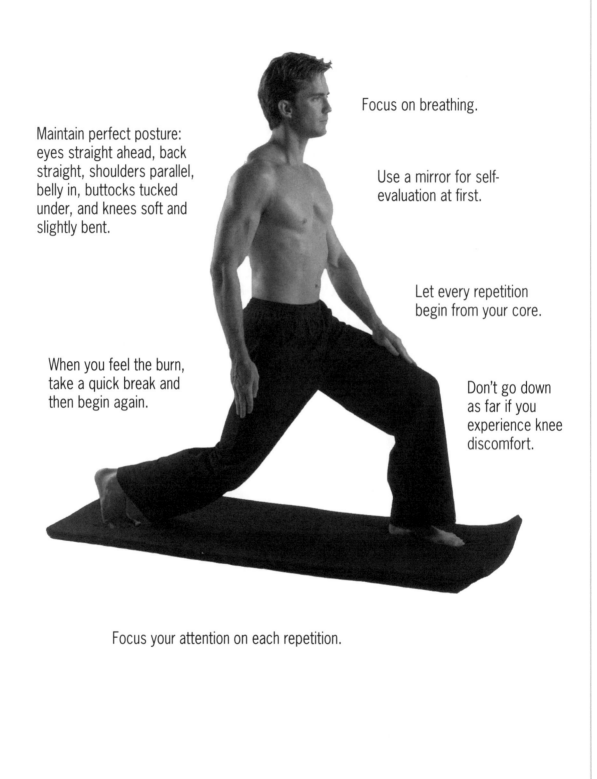

Maintain perfect posture: eyes straight ahead, back straight, shoulders parallel, belly in, buttocks tucked under, and knees soft and slightly bent.

Focus on breathing.

Use a mirror for self-evaluation at first.

Let every repetition begin from your core.

When you feel the burn, take a quick break and then begin again.

Don't go down as far if you experience knee discomfort.

Focus your attention on each repetition.

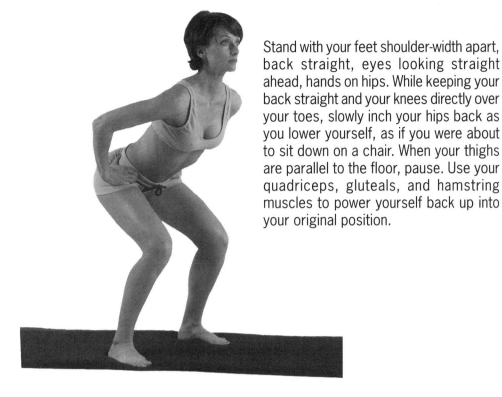

Stand with your feet shoulder-width apart, back straight, eyes looking straight ahead, hands on hips. While keeping your back straight and your knees directly over your toes, slowly inch your hips back as you lower yourself, as if you were about to sit down on a chair. When your thighs are parallel to the floor, pause. Use your quadriceps, gluteals, and hamstring muscles to power yourself back up into your original position.

# ONE-LEGGED DEAD LIFT

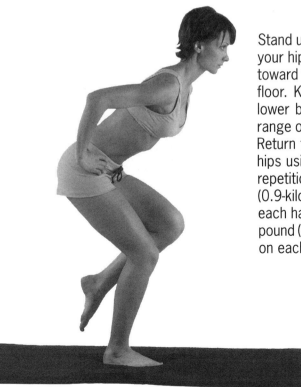

Stand upright on one leg with a slight bend in the knee, hands on your hips. Bend forward at the waist and slowly lower your torso toward the floor. The lifted leg remains bent, never touching the floor. Keep your head up, shoulders back, chest out, and the lower back in a flat position. Do not round the back. Limit the range of motion of the exercise to keep the back flat at all times. Return to the upright position by extending at the waist and the hips using the lower back and hamstring muscle groups. Do 10 repetitions with each leg. After a month, try holding a 2-pound (0.9-kilogram) dumbbell in each hand. Add 2 pounds a month to each hand until you can perform one-legged dead lifts with a 10-pound (4.5-kilogram) dumbbell in each hand. Maintain perfect form on each repetition.

# LUNGE

Hold your hands on your hips and take a slightly greater than normal step forward (slightly more than one foot, or 30 centimeters). Plant your lead foot and lower your body straight down until the trailing knee is just above the ground. Keep your torso upright, your back flat, and your knee in line with your foot. Return to the upright position by pushing off the lead leg to recruit your quadriceps and hip extensor muscles. Perform 10 repetitions with each leg. After a month, try holding a 2-pound (0.9-kilogram) dumbbell in each hand. Add 2 pounds a month to each hand until you can perform lunges with a 10-pound (4.5-kilogram) dumbbell in each hand. Maintain perfect form on each repetition.

# BACKWARD LUNGE

Place your hands on your hips and step backward with one leg. Rest only the ball of that foot on the ground. The stationary leg is the working leg. Simply squat straight down, using your stationary leg to support your body weight. Return to the start position using the quadriceps and hip extensors of the stationary leg. Perform 10 repetitions with each leg. After a month, try holding a 2-pound (0.9-kilogram) dumbbell in each hand. Add 2 pounds a month to each hand until you can perform lunges with a 10-pound (4.5-kilogram) dumbbell in each hand. Maintain perfect form on each repetition.

Place your hands on your hips and lunge forward with one leg. Do not return to the start position. Instead lunge forward with the other leg. Continue for 10 repetitions with each leg. After a month, try holding a 2-pound (0.9-kilogram) dumbbell in each hand. Add 2 pounds a month to each hand until you can perform lunges with a 10-pound (4.5-kilogram) dumbbell in each hand. Maintain perfect form on each repetition.

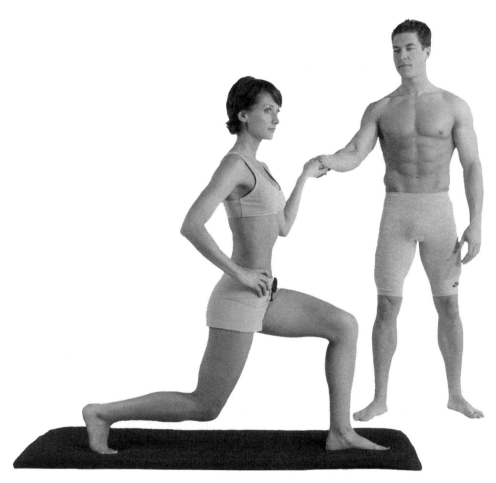

# SIDE LUNGE

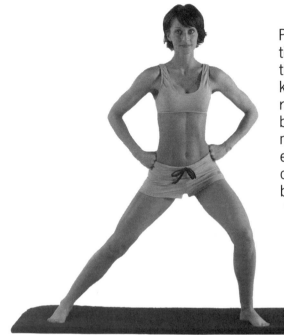

Place your hands on your hips and perform a combination of the squat and the lunge by stepping laterally. Plant the lead foot with your toes forward and squat. Keep the knees pointed over the toes. Push off the lead foot to return to the start position. Keep your torso upright and back flat. Perform 10 repetitions with each leg. After a month, try holding a 2-pound (0.9-kilogram) dumbbell in each hand. Add 2 pounds a month to each hand until you can perform lunges with a 10-pound (4.5-kilogram) dumbbell in each hand. Maintain perfect form on each repetition.

# ONE-LEGGED SQUAT

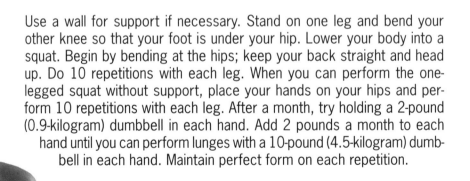

Use a wall for support if necessary. Stand on one leg and bend your other knee so that your foot is under your hip. Lower your body into a squat. Begin by bending at the hips; keep your back straight and head up. Do 10 repetitions with each leg. When you can perform the one-legged squat without support, place your hands on your hips and perform 10 repetitions with each leg. After a month, try holding a 2-pound (0.9-kilogram) dumbbell in each hand. Add 2 pounds a month to each hand until you can perform lunges with a 10-pound (4.5-kilogram) dumbbell in each hand. Maintain perfect form on each repetition.

# PROGRAMS

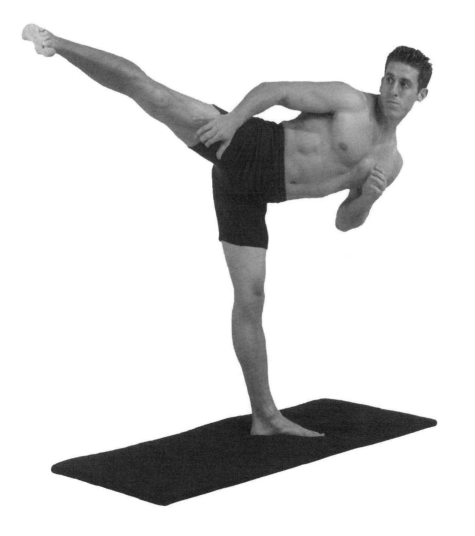

# part III

# COMPLETE TORSO CONDITIONING:

## Slimming and Toning

In our efforts to bring you the newest, most efficient forms of core training (and athletic abs), we have created a series of core drills (flexibility, martial arts, sports and plyometrics, kicking, and so on, done solo or with a training partner) that can affect your midsection (and whole body, for that matter) like nothing you have ever felt before. We later combine these drills into martial-arts-style katas (sequences of movements) with the sole purpose of ultimate ab development. Our drills are inspired by yoga, tai chi, kickboxing, taekwondo, krav maga, gymnastics, and more. Enjoy the variety as you learn more about your body and the infinite number of training possibilities.

# FLEXIBILITY DRILLS

We equate flexibility with awareness. A flexible body is one that, over time, becomes able to work throughout all ranges of motion without injury. We want you to increase your strength, flexibility, and awareness. The following exercises, although not stretches, help you do just that by enabling you to feel your range of motion without momentum and to focus on the muscles involved. Like slow-moving tai chi, these slow core-awareness exercises prepare you for the times when you need to move swiftly and instinctively in sport, exercise, or everyday life.

## From Tight to Flexible

When I was a 10-year-old Little League baseball player, I went to the doctor for my first physical (I hated that cough-to-the-right thing). When he asked me to touch my toes, I was able to get my fingertips only to just below my knees! He said, "Ooh, tight lower back." I came to understand that I was a bowlegged sprinter with tight shoulders inherited from my father and limited hamstring flexibility, which usually goes hand in hand with a tight lower back. Knowing these things, over the years I have been able to focus a little more on my quirks, and I am now proudly being touted as pretzel man at the local circus. Just kidding! But I am now able to bend over and place my hands flat on the floor. It is all workable.—Scott Cole

Standing with your feet slightly apart (shoulder-width or closer), extend both arms up over your head, inhaling as you lengthen your torso, arching naturally into your neutral spine position (a). Keep your knees slightly bent and your hips relaxed. Exhale as you lower your arms slowly, bending at the elbows as if pulling down on imaginary cables, contracting your abs, and squeezing the air out of your lungs like water out of a sponge (b). This drill is designed to get you to stretch, feeling the length of your abdominal muscles and the contraction on the return as well. Your easy breathing and your body awareness will greatly improve with this simple warm-up exercise. Perform at least five repetitions slowly.

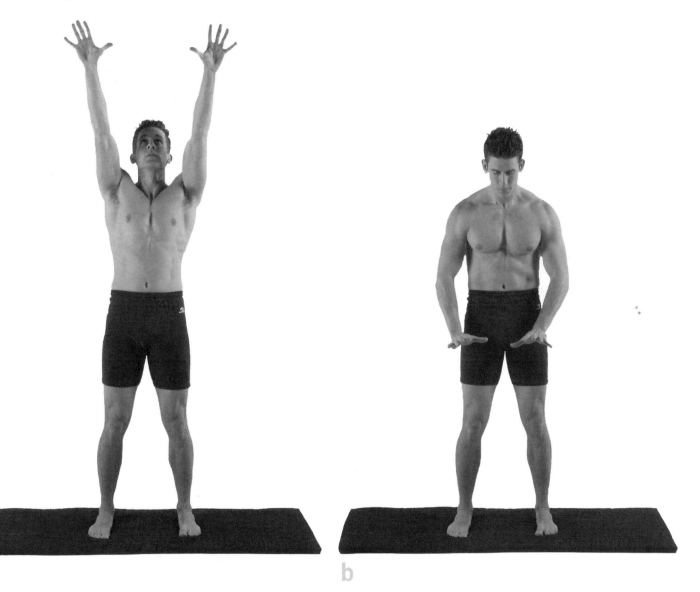

a

b

Like the elongated crunch, this is an awareness exercise without imposed resistance. Standing with your feet just a few inches apart, inhale and lift your right arm up slowly, bending slightly to the left as your arm reaches over your head (a). You should feel as though you are reaching up and out, rather than bending strangely sideways. Bend your left elbow and brace your left hand on your left hip. Keep your knees slightly bent as you exhale and bend the right elbow, pulling down on an imaginary cable, leaning into and activating the right side of your waist (b). Inhale as you reach over your head, feeling your side expand and lengthen through the range of motion. Exhale as you pull down, feeling the contraction. Perform at least five repetitions slowly, and repeat on the opposite side, always supporting your torso at the hip with the opposite arm.

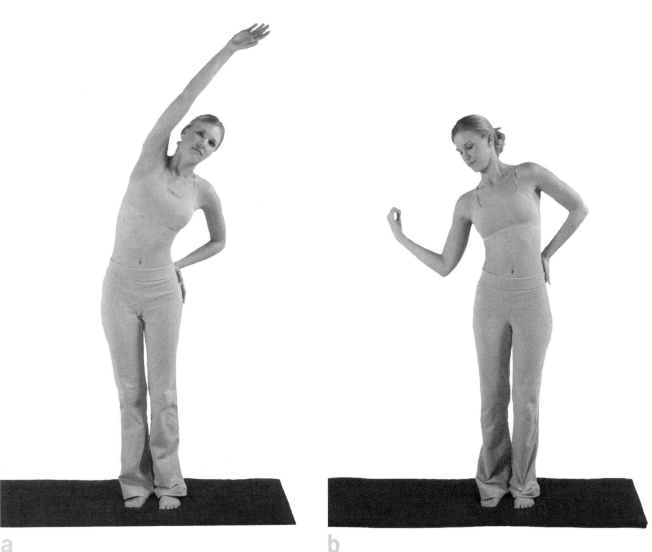

a

b

Stand with your feet slightly wider than shoulder-width apart in a modified horse stance, knees slightly bent, arms at your sides. Feel your centered core initiating movement as you reach out in front of you with your left arm, allowing your right shoulder, right arm, and torso to turn from the waist to the right, bending your right elbow to balance the movement (a). Staying centered in your strong leg base, reverse the movement slowly; then reach your right arm to the front, turning your torso to the left and bending your left elbow to balance the movement (b). It is important to focus, breathe, and not allow the movement to originate from tenseness in your shoulders. Allow the arm reach to be the by-product of relaxed energy from your core. You should feel the natural stability of the abs, obliques, and lower back as you perform the movement for 30 seconds to one minute, keeping your legs still and not shifting your weight forward or backward at all.

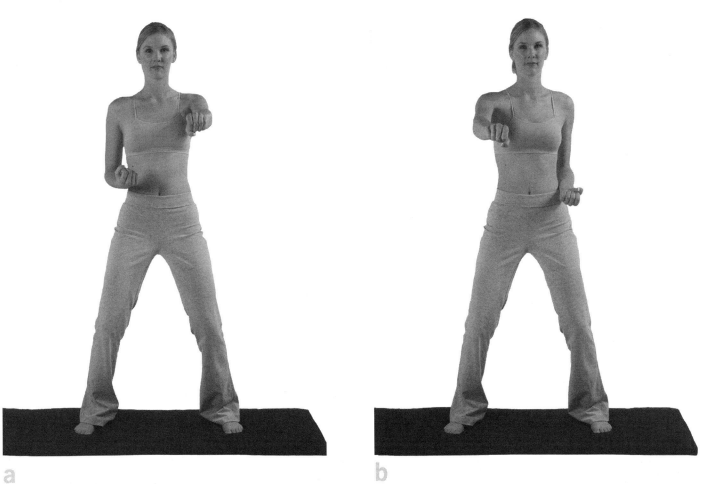

a

b

# MARTIAL ARTS DRILLS

Action drills initiated from the core have a martial arts quality that arises from feeling and understanding the origin of the movement. The martial arts quality is the centered awareness you feel as you move throughout the range of motion in the most energy-efficient, least-resistant way. If you are moving unconsciously (wasting your breath or flailing your limbs), you will feel the diminished results rather quickly because you will literally run out of energy. The more efficient your engine (your core), the stronger, more powerful, and sustained your activities will be. Relax into these exercises with a centered sense of power, and feel the results.

## Power From the Core

In the 1983 United States Taekwondo Championships, I fought future Olympic gold medalist Jimmy Kim. Kim absorbed my best shots to the body and countered with lethal spinning hook kicks. His counterattacks began from his core. The force of Kim's counterattacks knocked me to the floor even though they only struck my arms.

—Tom Seabourne

Stand with your feet slightly apart. March in place in slow motion, contracting your abdominal muscles naturally as you simultaneously raise your right knee so that your right foot leaves the floor, left arm moving forward with a bent elbow in opposition. Just before your right foot returns to the floor, raise your left knee in a simulated running motion, right arm following with a bent elbow. Focus on your abdominal muscles for a minute or so in slow motion. Now march in place in a relaxed fashion at a normal tempo, opposite arm and leg (just like walking), for one minute. Now run in place for two full minutes, knees and elbows moving in opposition (just like real running), your center of gravity lowered, focusing on your core connection.

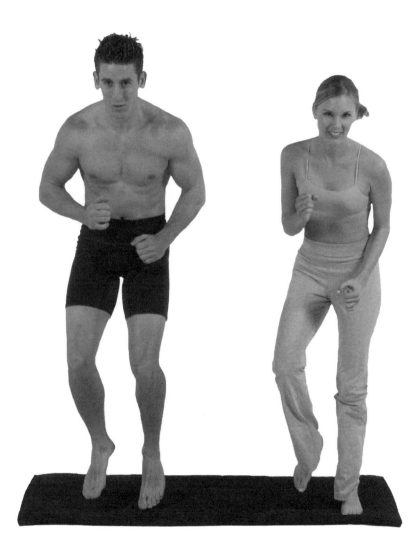

Begin in a horse stance with your feet a little more than shoulder-width apart and your knees slightly bent (a). Stand comfortably with your weight evenly distributed. Contract your left obliques by slowly turning your body to the right, staying centered, pivoting on the balls of your feet (b). This core-initiated action enables you to turn so that both feet point to the right at a 45-degree angle. Move slowly at first so that you know where you are going. Then, once you feel centered, alternate turning to the right and left (spine extended, not hunched over) and let a whiplike core effect commence. As you turn to the right, your right leg remains bent, and your left leg straightens slightly but with a soft knee; when you turn to the left, the left leg remains bent as the right straightens slightly. Repeat 10 times on both sides.

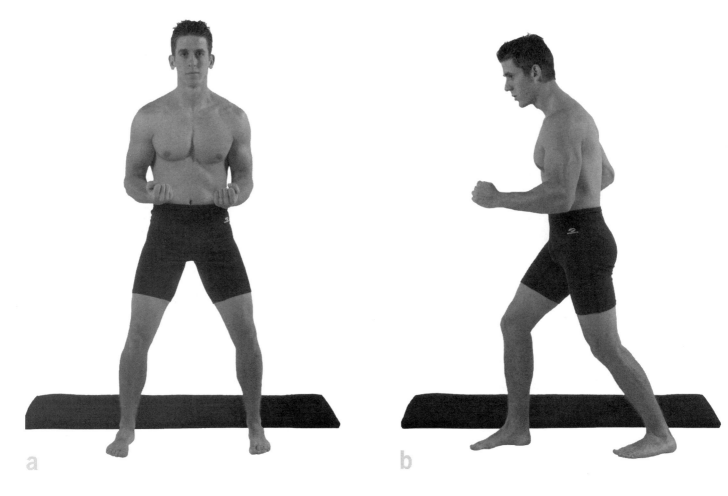

a

b

Begin in a square stance: your left foot points straight ahead and your right foot points directly to your right (a). Your feet are perpendicular so that you could trace a right angle that would intersect directly under your tailbone. Bend your knees over your toes and keep your weight evenly distributed. Contract your obliques as you simultaneously pivot on the ball of your right foot so that both feet are now pointed straight ahead (b). Your left knee remains bent while your right leg straightens slightly, but your knee is soft. Pivot back into a square stance, and repeat the square pivot with your other leg. As always, move slowly at first, so that your feet, knees, and hips are in alignment as you shift, allowing your core to really take charge. Perform 10 complete cycles (right, center, left, center is one cycle).

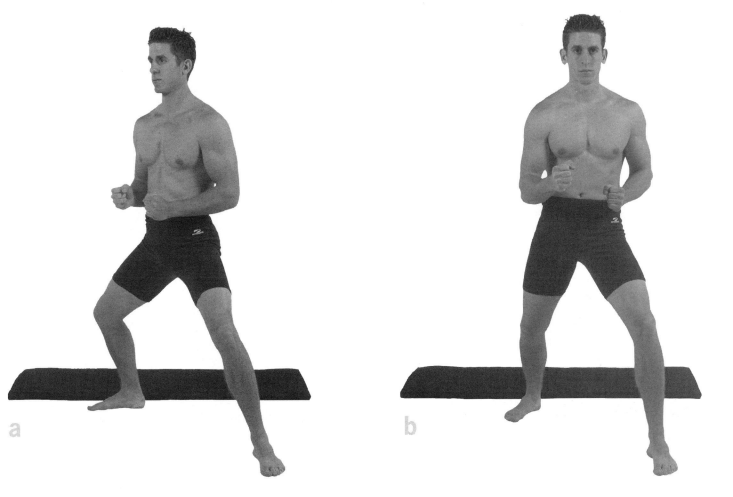

a

b

Begin in a square stance with your left foot pointing straight ahead and your right foot pointing directly to your right, contracting your abdominals with a slow exhalation (a). Pivot from a square stance to a front stance as you simultaneously contract each of the muscle groups in your torso, arms, and legs so that all the muscle groups in your entire body contract (b). Exhale slowly through pursed lips so that by the time you finish your exhalation, your pivot is complete and your core muscles are contracted. Move back into a square stance, take a deep breath, and repeat with your other leg. Add the opposing arm: as you shift to the left, the right arm follows with a flexed hand, and as you shift right, the left arm follows with a flexed hand. Keep your elbows close to your body, maintaining the "path of least resistance," feeling the centered power in your core. If you get all twisted up, you are not centered on your core and leg base. Perform at least 10 repetitions on each leg.

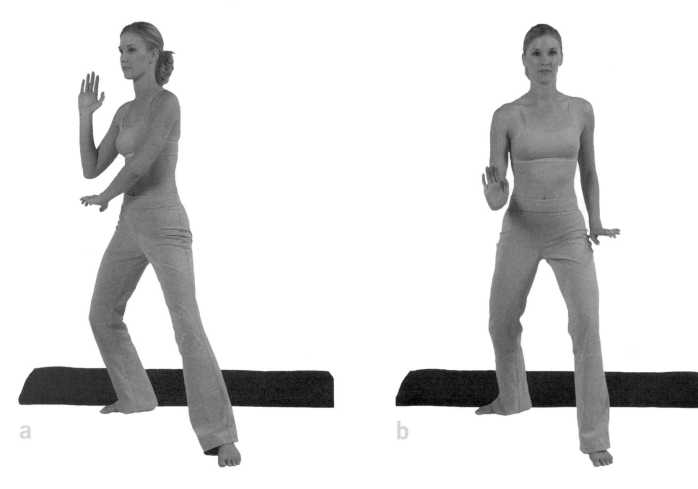

a                                     b

Like the brush push, this is a powerful core move, utilizing a surprising mixture of natural force. Stand with your weight on your right leg, right foot turned out for support. Your left foot is forward, perpendicular to the right foot, the ball touching and the heel up. Your right hand is up by your ear, your left arm is extended directly forward, palm up, over your left leg (a). Sit into your right leg, freeing your left leg, and step back diagonally onto your left foot, easing your weight onto the left leg (b). As you do, adjust your torso slightly to the left, right arm extending out now, left arm bending until the left hand is up by the ear or by the hip. Sit into it, feeling the rhythm of arms, legs, and core working together. Master it slowly, then try it fast, breathing with pursed lips, keeping your spine erect and elbows in close to your body. Unless you have a lot of space, you will have to step forward from time to time during this exercise since it moves diagonally backward. Do as many repetitions as you like slowly, then do at least 20, perhaps five sets of four, quickly and with awareness.

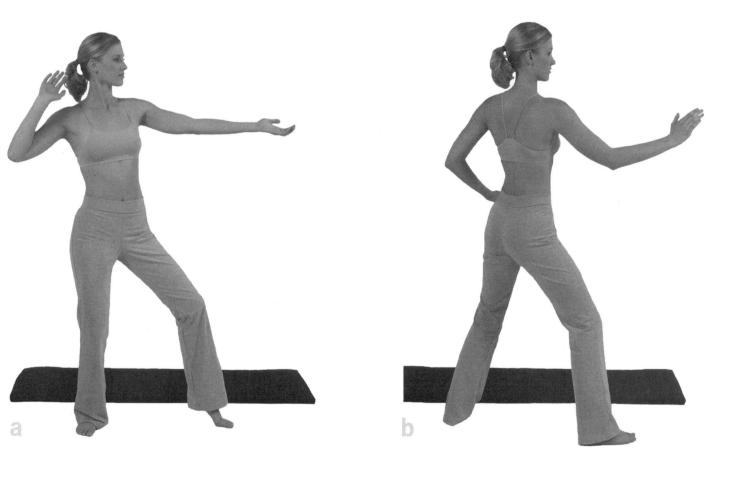

a     b

# SPORTS DRILLS AND PLYOMETRICS

Remember that power begins from your core. Punches, kicks, hits, or tosses are powered from your midsection. Plyometrics train your abs by providing a stretch, recoil, and then explosive movement through a full range of motion. For instance, in a jump, you feel the preparation, the extension, the bent-knee landing, and the potential explosive recoil from the landing. Plyometric drills can be performed with medicine balls, stability balls, and Thera-Bands, as well as with your own body and good, old-fashioned gravity.

Plyometric training is an excellent method for improving your core strength and power. You can also use plyometrics to train at a larger percentage of your aerobic capacity. Plyometrics are considered advanced training. If your knees, shins, hips, ankles, and back aren't in perfect condition, don't try these. Be sure you perform plyometrics on a soft surface, such as grass, a tartan track, or a floating wood or padded gymnastic floor.

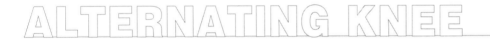

## ALTERNATING KNEE

Stand facing forward with your left foot slightly in front of your right foot. Keep your knees soft with your feet no more than shoulder-width apart. Raise your right knee forcefully, bringing your right foot up by your left knee, so that your left foot is actually pulled off the floor (a). Land gently on the floor on one foot then the other, rolling from the balls of your feet to your heels with your knees bent (b). Perform 10 times, switching legs. Once you master this, alternate legs for 20 repetitions.

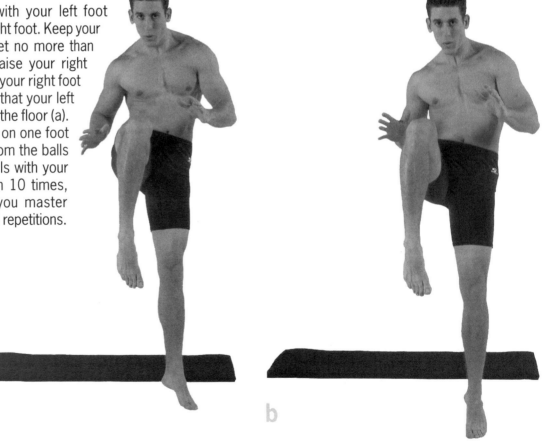

a                    b

Stand facing forward with your feet spread a few inches beyond shoulder-width. Lean to your left, pour your weight into your left leg, crouch with an extended spine, and slide your right leg toward your left leg so that the insteps of your feet almost touch (a). Bend your left knee so that it supports your body weight on the outside edge of your left foot as you now push sideways to the right, using the power from your left leg to propel you and sliding your right foot, right leg, torso, and arms to the right like a speed skater in motion (b). As you lean fully onto your right leg, slide your left foot toward your right leg so that the insteps of your feet almost meet. Continue this cycle for 10 repetitions, feeling the easy weight shift from leg to leg and the smooth resilience of your arms moving naturally with your legs, stabilized by your core.

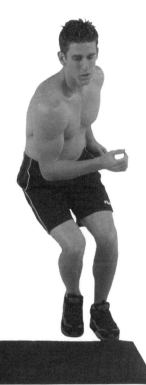

a

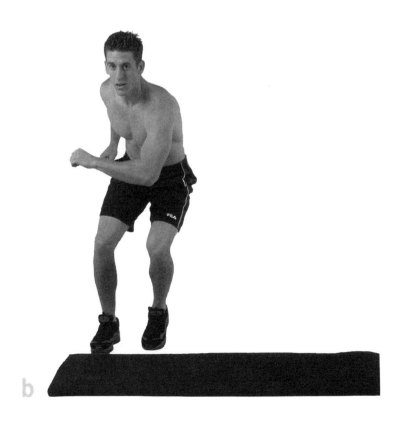

b

Around the clock is similar to the power slide except that you move in a variety of directions. Begin by facing forward with your feet spread a few inches beyond shoulder-width. Imagine that your left foot is at the 9 o'clock position (pm or am doesn't matter), and your right foot is at 3 o'clock. Slide your right foot over to your left so that all of your weight transfers to your left leg at 9 o'clock (a). Then slide your right foot over to the 3 o'clock position, shifting all of your weight to your right leg (b). Alternating legs, slide forward diagonally right to 1 o'clock, then back diagonally left to 7 o'clock. Take a small step over to 5 o'clock, slide forward diagonally left to 11 o'clock, right to 3 o'clock, left to 9 o'clock, and so on. Once you get the feel of this, you can play with slides in all directions, balancing right and left, forward and back, and the diagonals. Stay low into the quads, knees never extending beyond the toes. Breathe, keeping a relaxed sense of rhythm and strength.

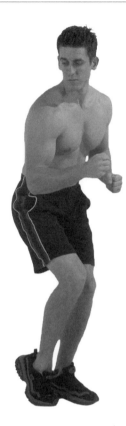

a

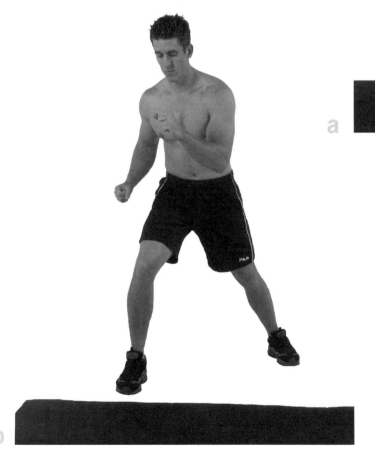

b

# PARTNER DRILLS

Each of these partner drills requires your abdominal muscles to stabilize your torso against the unexpected moves of your partner. These drills are a great way to train and to better understand your core and "gut instinct."

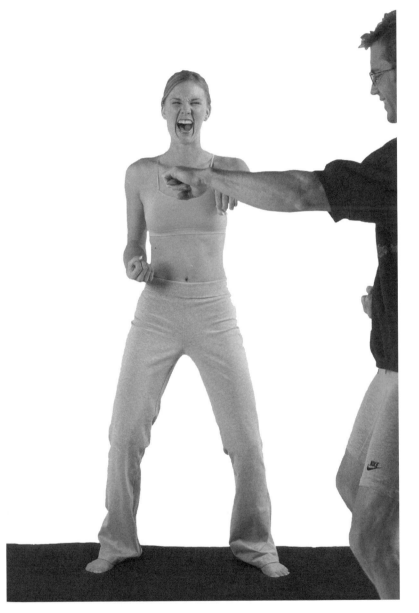

Partner drills are a great way to build your core strength. They're fun, too!

Stand with your feet slightly apart, arms relaxed at your sides. Allow your partner to lift you up from behind. You remain relaxed the first time, with no prior mental preparation. After your partner releases you, take a few seconds to center yourself, consciously dropping your energy and your weight into your hips, relaxing your entire body. Let your partner lift you again and feel the difference. You should seem "heavier" (not pound-wise, so don't panic) and feel more powerfully centered. Switch places and now lift your partner. This exercise reminds you how important it is to stay grounded in both your mental and physical activity.

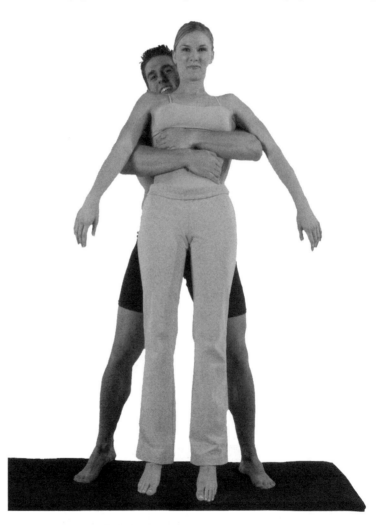

Face your partner and bow (might as well make it official). You should both step forward on the right foot, instep to instep. You both raise your right arms, elbows bent, shoulders relaxed, and touch each other at the back of the wrist. Keep this connection, feeling your partner's energy as you move slowly forward and back, bending at the ankles, knees, and hips, while turning at the waist. Try to minimize the arm movement, focusing on the stability of your core, allowing your arms to follow the strength of your core and the turning of your waist. Although your legs move forward and back, your feet are planted at all times. Your torso rotates in a circular motion because of the turning at your waist and the activation of your core. Stay connected, changing the direction of your circle. Then switch legs, connecting at the back of the left wrist this time, and repeat the circular movement in both directions. Breathe, and stay relaxed, allowing your body to really open up.

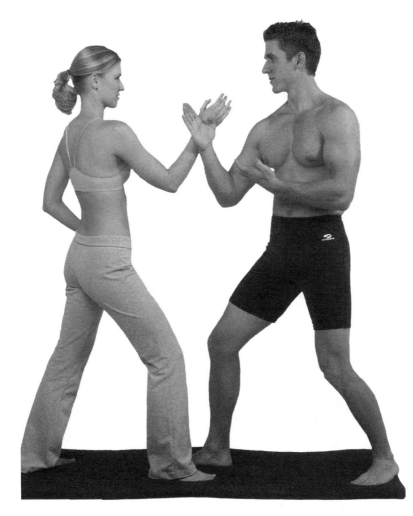

Stand facing your partner. Both of you should stand with your left foot forward, your elbows in, and your hands up. Maintain light contact with your partner's hands, moving them in a circular motion. Be sure there is no unnecessary muscular contraction as you allow your hands to flow in a circular pattern without thought or intent. Once this circular flow becomes automatic, attack your partner (playfully, of course, but with intent) by trying to make contact with his or her body with one of your hands. Your partner's response should be to deflect your hand while maintaining the perfect flow of the circle. Any muscular effort or sharp movement should be avoided. After one minute, allow your partner to attack you. Deflect his or her strikes with an almost effortless intensity generated from your constantly contracted core. After one minute, you both attack and defend at will. Block and attack with no thought. After that, close your eyes and continue blocking and attacking for another minute, feeling the strength of deflection and a well-centered core.

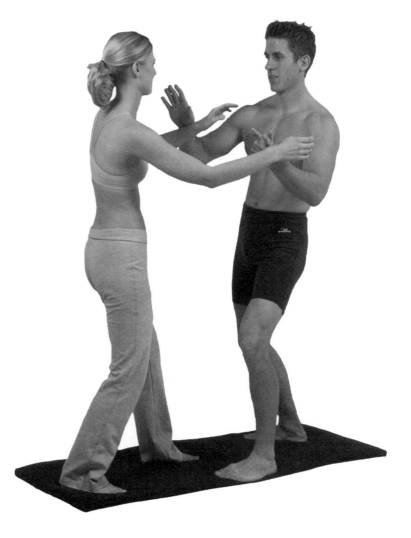

Stand facing your partner with your hands up and your elbows close to your body. Gently touch your partner with your first two knuckles on your partner's abdomen, establishing a contact point. Your partner's response should be an immediate pursed-lip exhalation, forcing the abdominal muscles to contract. Bring your hands back up, and allow your partner to gently strike you. Contract your abdominal muscles. Continue trading punches to all areas of your abdomen for two minutes. Have fun with it, using your legs as a strong base, feeling the stability in your core, and utilizing the power of your breath as a training tool.

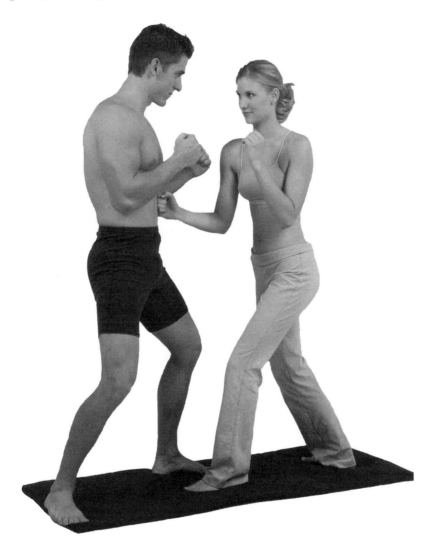

# INDIVIDUAL KICK DRILLS

You may be wondering why kicks are included in an abdominal program. Strong legs, strong core, big power, and stability beyond any kind of compartmentalized abdominal training is the answer. If you think kicking involves only the legs, wait until you see the increase in your overall flexibility by doing these kick drills. If you are skeptical, we'll laugh with you (not at you) as you really feel your core muscles the day after performing these drills. Relax into your center, and have fun with these.

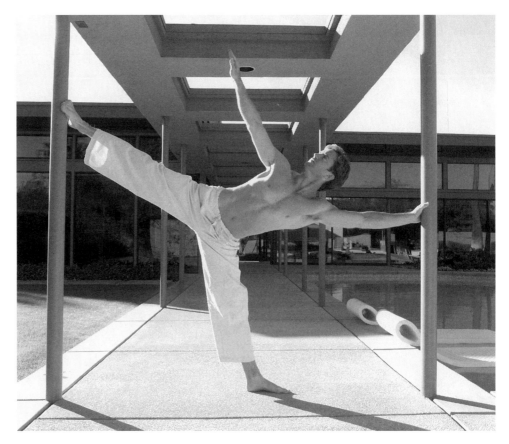

Kicking involves more than just the legs. Kick drills increase flexibility and power your core.

Your core controls your movement. At first, hold on to a wall for balance. As you grow stronger and your balance improves after many training sessions, you will rely on the wall less and less. Within six months, you will not need the wall at all.

**Step 1:** Hold on to a wall for balance. Practice slow, controlled leg swings to the front, side, and back. Perform 10 repetitions with each leg for each direction.

**Step 2:** Perform leg swings as in step 1, but instead of letting your leg drop right away, hold it at maximum height for three seconds.

**Step 3:** Hold your leg up in an isometric position for three seconds. Use every ounce of your strength to keep your leg from dropping. Attempt to hold the position with leg strength alone for three seconds, then relax.

**Step 4:** Perform the leg swings without using the wall. Be conscious of contracting your abdominal muscles and stabilizing your pelvis to maintain perfect posture.

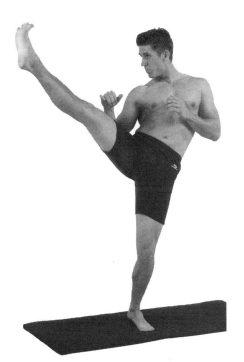

front

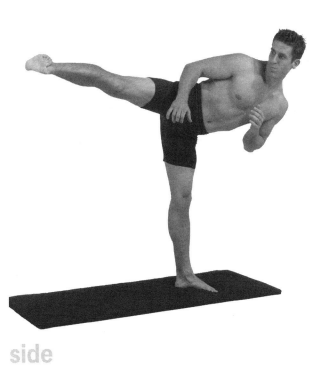

side

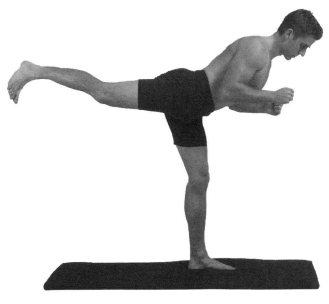

back

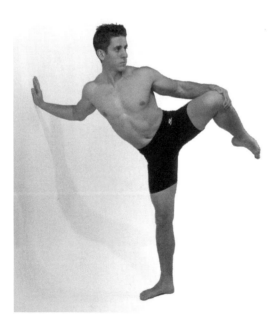

For a roundhouse kick fold position, hold the inside of your left knee parallel to the floor and your knee flexed. The position resembles a puppy standing beside a fire hydrant getting ready to do his business.

**Step 1:** Hold a wall for balance with your right hand. Lift your left leg up to your side in a roundhouse kick fold position.

**Step 2:** Use your left hand to raise your knee a little higher. Then let go with your hand and attempt to keep your knee up using the strength of your core.

**Step 3:** Perform 10 consecutive roundhouse kick folds. Switch sides and repeat.

**Step 4:** Perform this exercise without using the wall. Be conscious of contracting your abdominal muscles and stabilizing your pelvis to maintain perfect posture.

step 1

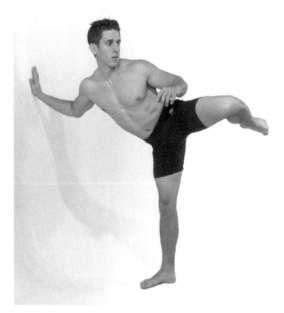

step 2a

step 2b

The hook kick moves in the opposite direction of a roundhouse kick. It comes around from the back.

**Step 1:** Hold on to a wall with your left hand. Lift your right knee into a hook kick-fold position.

**Step 2:** Use your right hand to add a few more inches of height.

**Step 3:** Do 10 consecutive side hook kicks without allowing your knee to drop. Switch sides and repeat.

**Step 4:** Perform this exercise without using the wall. Be conscious of contracting your abdominal muscles and stabilizing your pelvis to maintain perfect posture.

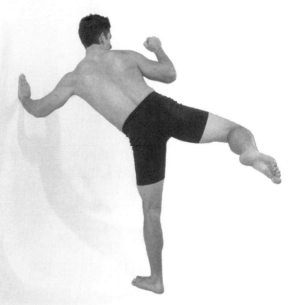

step 1

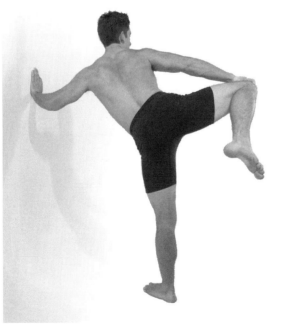

step 2

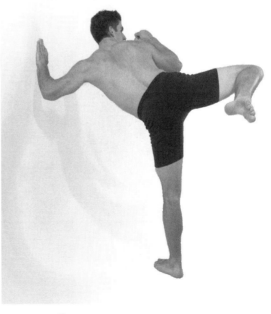

step 3

## PARTNER FLOOR DRILLS

Partners can help stabilize each other for amazing strength, flexibility, and motivational gains. The following two exercises can also be done individually with the help of a chair and some imagination.

## TIGHT-BODY DRILL (TWO LEGS, ONE LEG)

Lie flat on your back, legs and feet together, arms at your sides, palms facing down. Your partner lifts your feet off the ground while you try to maintain a straight body by using core strength (a). It requires control of the hips, legs, and abs to keep your body in a straight position with only your shoulders and arms touching the ground. (Your arms are at your sides for balance and support; try not to push into the ground with your arms.) Your partner should not lift you beyond 45 degrees. Talk to each other; maintain relaxed breathing. Once you are comfortable with the two-legged version, have your partner let go of one foot, requiring you to balance with only one leg supported (b). Explore the drill: switch legs, go back to two, then to one, strengthening your core all the while. Be nice to your partner, though, because you have to switch.

The tight-body drill can be done individually by placing your feet (heels and Achilles tendons) on a chair. A level 1, or beginning, exerciser can put the lower legs up to the backs of the knees entirely on the chair. The more of your body you put on the chair, the easier the drill becomes.

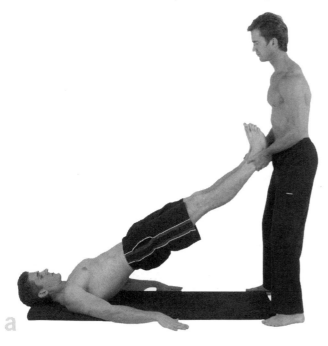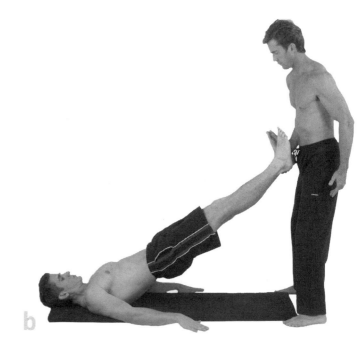

Lie on your back with your hands up, protecting your face. Your knees should be bent with your feet flat on the floor. Your partner stands in front of you and moves from side to side and around you, as if trying to attack (a). Your goal is to keep your feet between you and your partner by shuffling your feet from side to side, moving your body around, spinning on your back like a top, or turning in a full circle if required. Occasionally, your partner should do a bluff move in toward you. Counter this movement with a kick toward your opponent (b), either forward or to the side (turn quickly onto your side as your partner feints). The attacking partner needs to be careful to keep a 12-inch (30-centimeter) margin of error in all attacks and defenses. (In other words, avoid making contact, and give your crab some space!) Feel your core in a slightly curled, contracted position. Notice that if you tighten up, you are slower and less effective on the ground. Be ready for any movement by staying relaxed. Relaxing gives you more speed, more endurance, and much more power in your kicks. Trade places after one minute, and continue with four more cycles.

This exercise can be done without a partner. Just imagine a partner coming at you from all angles and go with it, just like shadow boxing (minus the shadow).

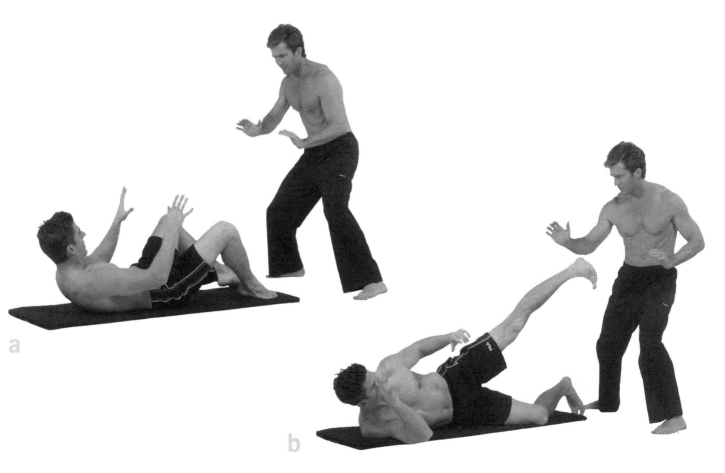

a

b

# YOGA-INSPIRED INDIVIDUAL FLOOR DRILLS

Yoga-inspired exercises are hard to beat when it comes to integrating flexibility and power. These exercises balance your muscles by involving the abs, back, obliques, and more. Remember to breathe, go for your natural range of motion, and stay centered.

## CAT BACK

Get on all fours, knees below the hips, hands below the shoulders, elbows slightly bent, with your back flat, similar to a tabletop. Inhale and allow gravity to arch your back naturally as you stretch gently through your abs (a). Once expanded, perform the reverse arch by bringing your navel toward your spine, exhaling, and rounding and stretching your back as you bring your chin toward your chest (b). Hold that position for a comfortable second and repeat, maintaining an easy breathing rhythm and the flow of a moving meditation. Do 10 repetitions, really feeling your breath and the symbiotic relationship between your abs and your back muscles.

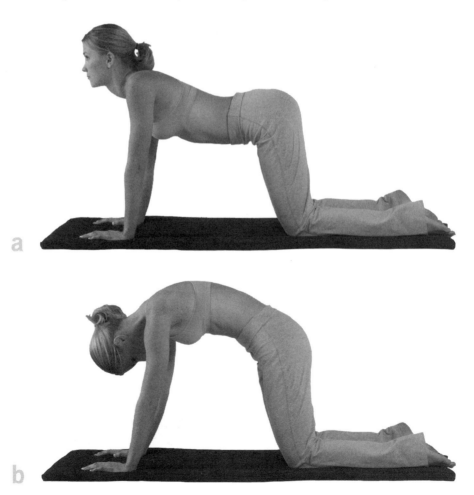

It is time for some strong, lengthened fun. Again in neutral position on all fours, with knees in a little closer, brace yourself with your right foot flexed (toes braced on the floor). Bend your left knee in, and extend your left leg fully parallel to the floor (a). Now, extend your right arm out in front of you, biceps by the ear, palm slightly turned up to relax the shoulder (b). Breathe, balancing with your core and feeling the length of the posture.

For variation, curl your left leg to a 90-degree hamstring curl with a flexed foot, extend your right arm out to the side with palm down, hold a few seconds, then extend your leg out again parallel to the floor, point your foot, return your arm to the extended position (biceps by the ear), then slowly come down to all fours.

Notice whether you are out of breath. Many people try too hard and forget to breathe. Now relax, shake it out, and do the other side. Left foot flexed, toes to the floor, right leg extends out, pointed foot, left arm extends out, bicep to ear (if you can extend your right arm, you will set a new human record), flexed foot now, hamstring curl, arm variation out to your side, palm down, extended leg again, pointed foot, arm returns to original position, and down. Breathe and move on.

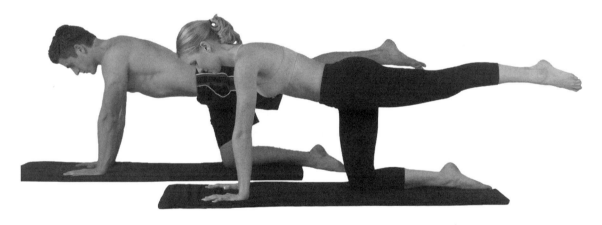

a

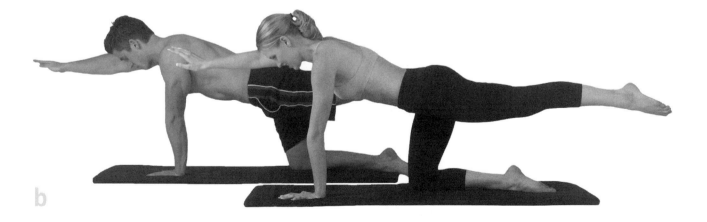

b

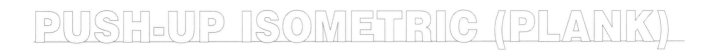

Move now into a push-up position (oh, joy!). Support yourself on your knees if on your toes is too much for you. Push-ups train stabilizer muscles in your back and abdomen, as well as working your chest and triceps. When performing push-ups, your head and neck remain neutrally aligned due to the isometric contraction of your cervical spine. The abdominals, erector spinae (back) muscles, hip flexors (the muscles that lift the leg, hip to knee), and glutes (buttocks) all contract, stabilizing your body, holding you safely in the push-up position, and preventing your hips from sinking to the floor. Breathe naturally, maintaining the lengthened strength position, never locking your elbows. Then try balancing on one foot only, switch back to two, and so on, trying not to shake or to vary or compromise your position. Feel your core working to keep your body balanced and in alignment.

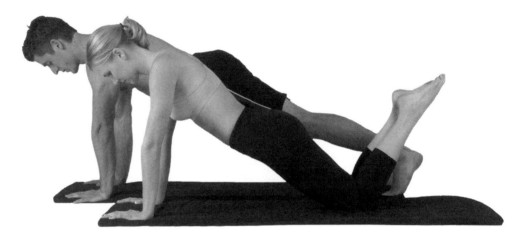

Start in an abdominal stretch, lying on your belly, forearms on the ground, chest lifted, and shoulders relaxed (a). Curl your toes under in a flexed foot position, and slowly lift the hips and pelvis off the floor out of the modified cobra pose and into a straight-line position (b). A proper plank is performed on the floor with your hands either a little less than shoulder-width or together in the "triangle arm" position; your elbows are below your shoulders with forearms resting on the floor in either hand position. Keep your arms in close to your body and your back straight with a slight arch in your lower spine. Your neck supports your head in a neutral position. The plank (an isometric contraction) works virtually every muscle and requires strength and stamina to hold for prolonged periods of time. Don't worry, we are not recommending substituting your lunch break for a held plank, but we want you to get strong enough to challenge yourself to 15 seconds and then 30 seconds. Breathe, of course, and alternate from the original position to a single leg for five seconds, back to center for five seconds, then onto the other leg for five seconds. Do not compromise your form on any of these exercises.

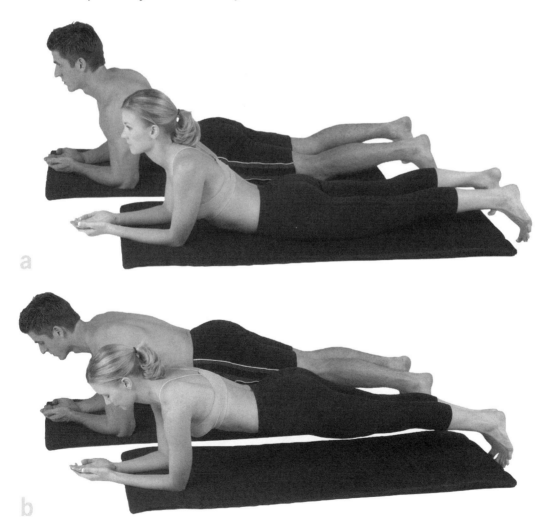

a

b

This one requires concentration and flexibility. Lie on your right side, braced on your right elbow, with your ankles crossed (left over right) and your feet off the ground, right outer thigh touching the floor (a). Roll over, switching sides and positions, so that your left side and left outer thigh touch the floor now and your ankles cross the other way (right over left) (b). Ease into each position, bringing your knees in toward your chest as you roll onto your back during the important transition between positions. Feel free to rest your head on your free hand as you become more coordinated with the movement. You will feel this full-body and core conditioning immediately. Do this exercise slowly until you master the movement, then speed it up to a comfortable drill pace. Remember, though, to keep it muscle based, not momentum based.

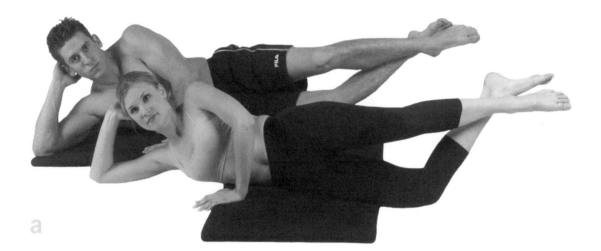

a

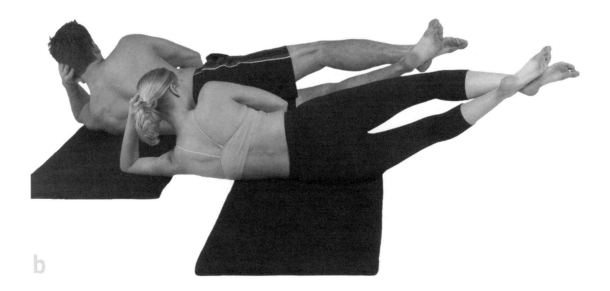

b

# FLOOR CORE KATA

A martial artist feels the movement of his or her body. Our goal with the floor core kata is to bring home the value of nonlinear training. Athletic abs are not achieved by just doing a set of moves. Intensity, focus, and technique really add to the experience and improve results. As you become more familiar with these exercises, your body will naturally hold the steady positions longer and transition between exercises with more grace and muscular control. You will experience multidimensional stability and the benefits of a strong core.

## Key Points for the Floor Core Kata

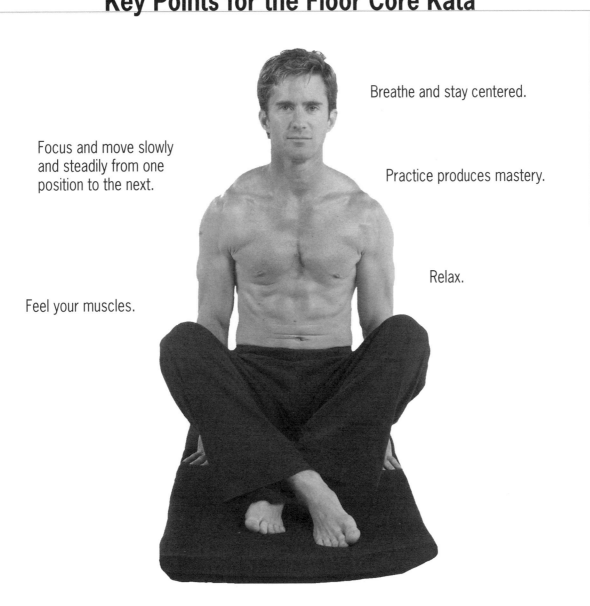

Breathe and stay centered.

Focus and move slowly and steadily from one position to the next.

Practice produces mastery.

Relax.

Feel your muscles.

Begin in a seated balance. For starters, sit cross-legged, knees bent and arms slightly bent with your hands flat on the floor. Lift your hips off the ground using your triceps and your abdominals. Your arms straighten as you lift your hips. Breathe as you hold the position for 5 to 10 seconds. Relax. Repeat two more times. For the advanced version, now try lifting your feet off the ground as you press up.

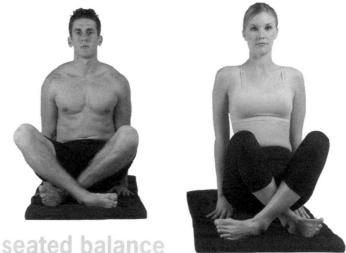

seated balance

Ease down back to the seated cross-legged position. From the seated position, uncross your legs, knees bent and feet out front, flat on the ground about shoulder-width apart. Lean your torso slightly backwards, resting in front of your tailbone (not right on it); stabilize with your hip flexors and core muscles as you lift your feet off the ground, knees still bent, stabilizing in your core. Circle your feet outward four times, then inward four times. Arms are open, palms up, not touching your legs. Breathe, stay centered, point your toes. Cross the right ankle over the left, then cross the left ankle over the right, then bring your feet and legs together.

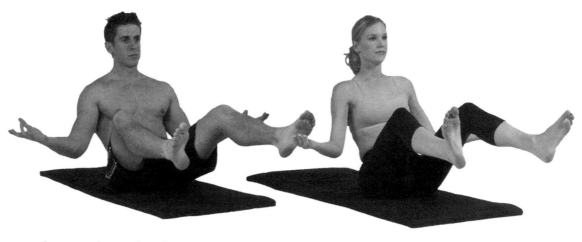

lean back, legs up

Extend your legs slowly into a V-sit (legs piked out front), then relax and slowly lower the legs. You may feel shaky, but with a little practice, you will be able to perform this sequence easily.

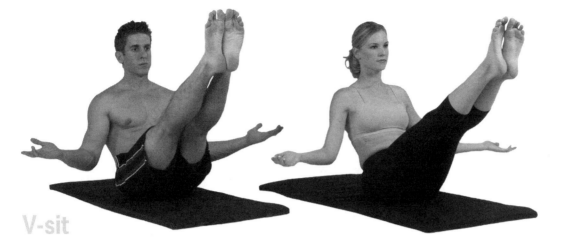

V-sit

After you master the first sequence, bring in other floor elements.

After your extended V-sit, roll sideways into the roll-over obliques, performing five slow, complete repetitions on each side.

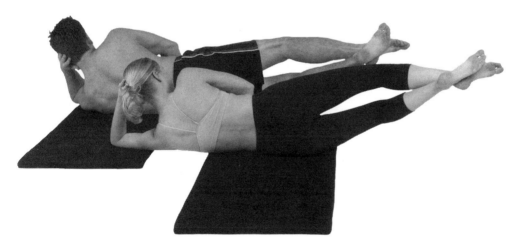

roll-over obliques

Extend your legs out in front of you in a 90-degree seated position, fingertips pointing away from your body, palms down. Ease up into a reverse tabletop: hands and feet are flat on the ground, torso and hips lifted up toward the sky, neck naturally in line with the spine, face looking up. Your shins and arms should be parallel to each other and perpendicular to the floor. Your feet can be shoulder-distance apart or together. Try this position with fingertips facing toward your body and then away from your body. Breathe, holding the posture for 10 seconds, then lower. Put your feet and legs together and go back up into the reverse tabletop position, pelvis toward the sky. Hold again for 10 seconds (the position, not your breath).

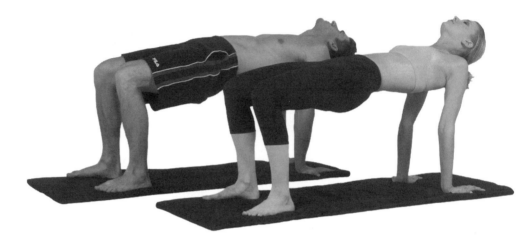

reverse tabletop

Extend into three more sets of roll-over obliques. After the last repetition, turn over into the push-up isometric, or plank, position. Hold this position for five seconds, then ease your way slowly down and up through five complete push-ups. Modify by using the knee push-up position if necessary.

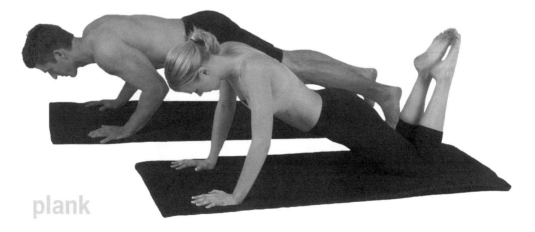

plank

Ease down, chest to floor, hands at shoulder level. With your forearms on the floor, raise your chest slowly into the modified cobra, curling your toes under for support as you ease into the forearm plank.

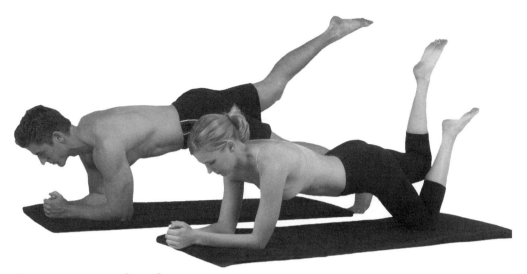

forearm plank

Hold the forearm plank position for 10 seconds. Then repeat using the right leg only for five seconds, both legs again for five seconds, left leg for five seconds, both again for five seconds, then down, rolling over onto your back for an individual krav maga crab drill.

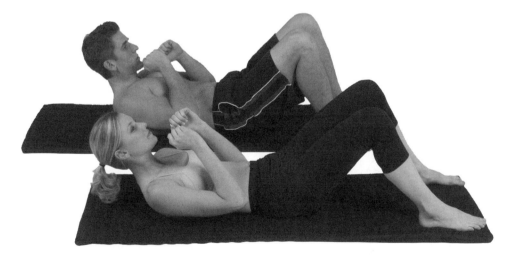

krav maga crab

COMPLETE TORSO CONDITIONING: Slimming and Toning

On your back, knees and elbows bent, feet touching the floor, abs curled, and hands up near your face, perform the individual krav maga crab drill for at least 30 seconds, shuffling your feet to the right, then the left, then center. Roll onto your right side to perform a quick left side kick, then back to center, then to the other side. Play with it, testing your core at all angles. Relax back, stretch your arms overhead, lengthen out, and then make your way to all fours.

On all fours, stretch your abs and your back with the yoga cat back, breathing naturally, taking your time, feeling the extension of the spine, as if performing a slow-moving meditation. Maintain this pose until you feel sufficiently slowed down and your heart rate is back to normal (one or two minutes or so).

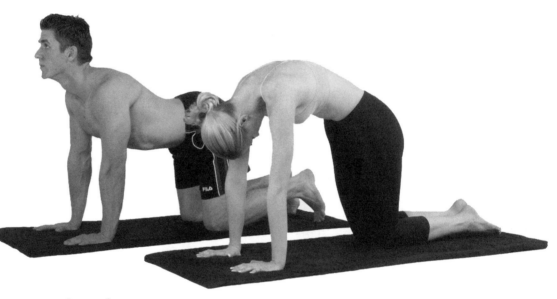

cat back

Ease into a forward bend, knees bent, buttocks to heels, arms extended forward, fingertips spread, hands and forehead on the floor. If you are comfortable, ease back all the way into the child's pose (see chapter 2), breathing deeply, relaxing, and stretching your whole body, especially your lower back.

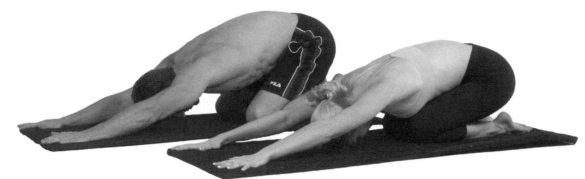

forward bend

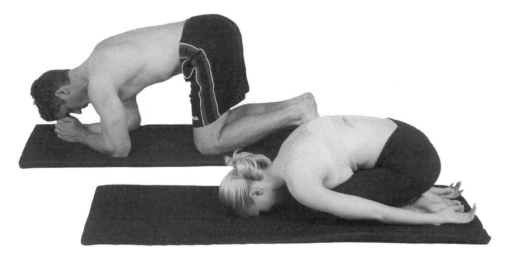

child's pose

# Advanced Moves

More advanced students can eventually perform the piked press or straddle press.

For the piked press, sit in a 90-degree pike sit, legs straight out in front of you, feet together, with your hands on the ground, leaning slightly forward from your hips. Your goal is to lift your legs and hips off the ground while maintaining the piked position with your legs. Your hands are the only point of contact with the ground. Gymnasts often perform this move on the floor, on parallel bars, or on the rings.

The straddle press requires similar core strength as the piked press except your legs are in the open or straddle position. Sitting with your hands on the floor, lift your hips, butt, legs, and feet so your hands are the only point of contact with the ground. Hands can be placed between your legs or on the sides of your hips.

These moves illustrate why gymnasts have some of the best abs on earth.

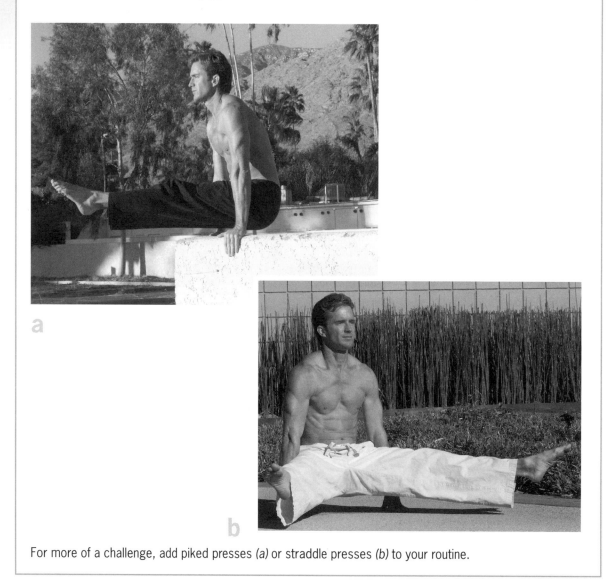

a

b

For more of a challenge, add piked presses (a) or straddle presses (b) to your routine.

# STANDING CORE KATA

Your core power is generated from your legs and hips. A strong base of support aids your core training. When you strike or kick a ball, an equal force is generated in both directions. To hit through a target, you must shift your weight and relax into a rock-solid stance. Your whole body is involved in these movements. The standing core kata will fortify your core from the ground up. At first, hold each stance for three seconds before proceeding to the next stance. Add two seconds each week until you can maintain each position for 30 seconds. Perform stance training at least three days per week.

## Key Points for the Standing Core Kata

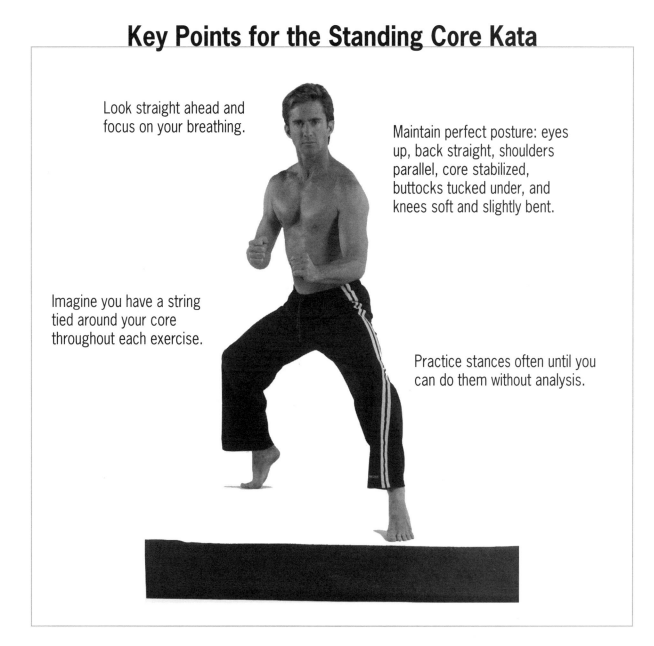

Look straight ahead and focus on your breathing.

Maintain perfect posture: eyes up, back straight, shoulders parallel, core stabilized, buttocks tucked under, and knees soft and slightly bent.

Imagine you have a string tied around your core throughout each exercise.

Practice stances often until you can do them without analysis.

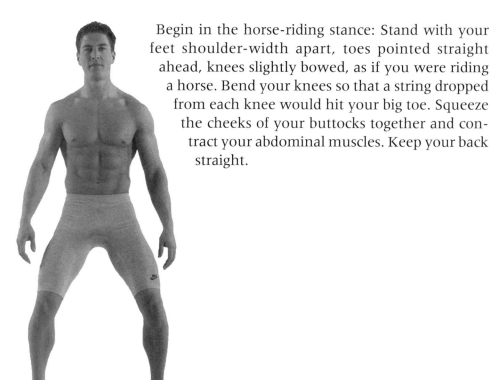

Begin in the horse-riding stance: Stand with your feet shoulder-width apart, toes pointed straight ahead, knees slightly bowed, as if you were riding a horse. Bend your knees so that a string dropped from each knee would hit your big toe. Squeeze the cheeks of your buttocks together and contract your abdominal muscles. Keep your back straight.

horse-riding stance

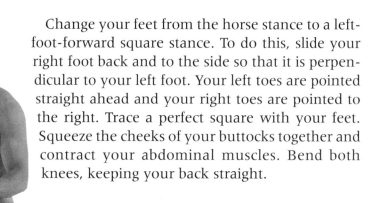

Change your feet from the horse stance to a left-foot-forward square stance. To do this, slide your right foot back and to the side so that it is perpendicular to your left foot. Your left toes are pointed straight ahead and your right toes are pointed to the right. Trace a perfect square with your feet. Squeeze the cheeks of your buttocks together and contract your abdominal muscles. Bend both knees, keeping your back straight.

square stance

Stand in a square stance and raise your heels off the floor. This exercise is good muscular endurance training for your upper and lower legs. It is outstanding for the calves. Squeeze the cheeks of your buttocks together and contract your abdominal muscles.

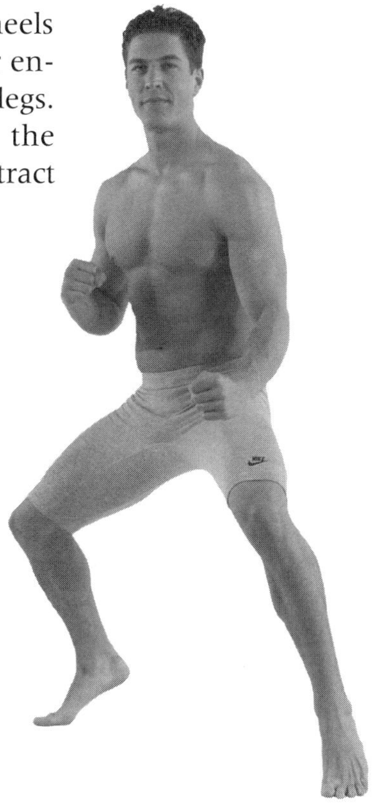

raise heels

Lower heels to the floor. Pivot into a front stance so that your right leg is forward and your right knee is bent. Transfer your weight to your right leg as you lean sideways. Squeeze the cheeks of your buttocks together and contract your abdominal muscles. Switch legs by placing your left foot forward and bending your left knee and repeat.

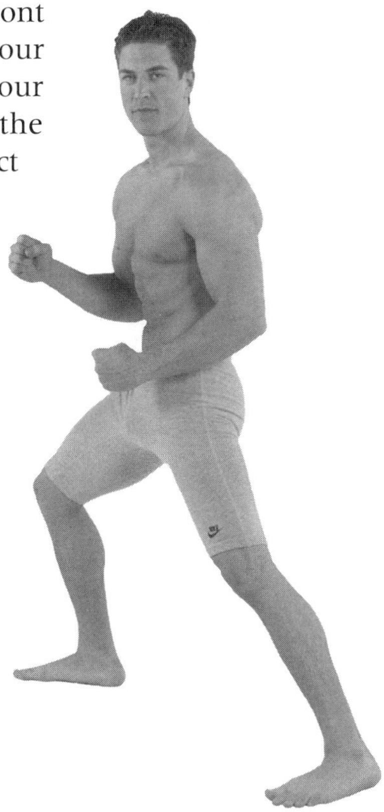

front stance

Change to a front stance with your left leg back and your right leg forward. Bend your right knee over your toe and lift your left leg off the floor toward the back. Keep the back leg straight. Continue to balance with your left leg in the air and your weight over the right knee. Contract the abdominal muscles and the gluteals of the back leg. Your back toes point down to the ground; your arms are open for balance. Flex and point your rear foot as you hold the leg position without wavering. Switch legs and repeat.

**balance**

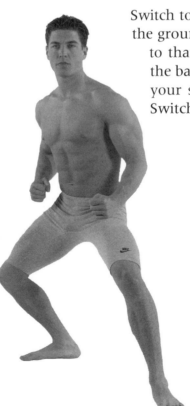

Switch to a cat stance by lowering your back leg to the ground and shifting 70 percent of your weight to that leg. Balance the rest of your weight on the ball of your front foot. Contract the glutes of your supporting leg, stabilizing with your abs. Switch legs and repeat.

**cat stance**

Assume a front stance with your left leg forward. Bend your right knee so that it comes within one inch (2.5 centimeters) of the floor. Imagine that you have a string tied around your waist. Switch legs and repeat.

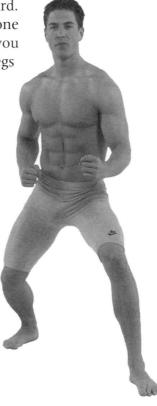

front stance, lower knee

Stand in a horse stance with your feet shoulder-width apart and toes turned inward. (This is called an hourglass stance.) Hold the position with strong abs.

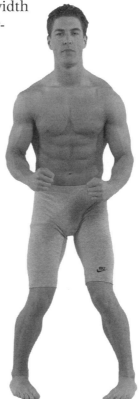

hourglass stance

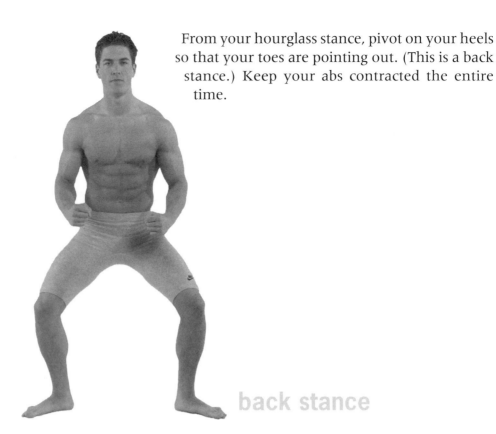

From your hourglass stance, pivot on your heels so that your toes are pointing out. (This is a back stance.) Keep your abs contracted the entire time.

back stance

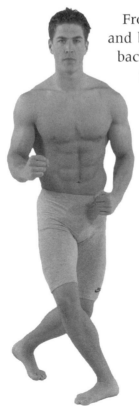

From your back stance, cross one leg behind the other and bend both knees. Take one step to the right, come back to center, then take one step to the left. Keep your toes pointed straight ahead. Your knees are bent throughout the exercise. Your head and shoulders remain parallel as you travel back and forth. Your abs should remain contracted through the duration of the exercise.

traveling

Stand with your feet close together and your heels spread apart. Lift your heels off the floor as you rise up on the balls of your feet. Make it a point to contract your abdominal muscles.

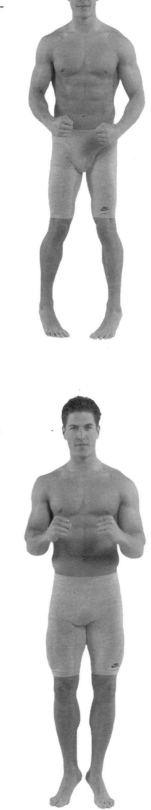

lift heels

Touch your heels together as you rise up on the balls of your feet. Keep your abdominal muscles firm and contracted.

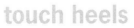

touch heels

# 10

# BODYBUILDING:
## Muscles for Power

Learn to beautifully master your body by continually strengthening your core. The exercises in this chapter stabilize your spine, shoulder girdle, and pelvic area so that all of your muscles can handle more weight and grow larger. Increasing your core strength makes you stronger and more efficient because your body parts are working in total synchronization. With core strength, your system is balanced so that no single muscle group becomes overloaded. You might not yet believe or understand how your arms and legs can actually grow in size by strengthening your core through these drills, but they will. Your strong torso balances with your upper and lower limbs, allowing better training. This chapter focuses on intense sports training, medicine ball drills, and plyometric training.

Your body can adapt to anything. We want you to grow and change, reaching higher as you see results. This program offers constantly varying stimuli to induce continuous adaptation. You will be amazed at how fast you will improve on these programs. We will keep you hopping between stability balls, medicine balls, and body-weight resistance. This program is about varying your time on task—sometimes to improve your muscular endurance and other times to enhance your absolute strength.

Medicine balls help you to train your torso at every angle and speed. Medicine balls come in all different weights, colors, and sizes. At first, begin with a light, small ball, one you can easily handle for every drill. Think of it this way: You control the ball, the ball should not control you.

Medicine balls can also train your nervous system to help you explode through a movement using plyometrics (plus you'll have a big new word to use at parties). Plyometrics help stimulate your fast-twitch muscle fibers. You can train with your medicine ball anywhere, and your results will be apparent in about a month. Train with your ball twice a week for best results.

## STANDING EXERCISES

Many people can't believe that standing exercises can be effective ab exercises. Always keep in mind that your core is the liaison between your arms and your legs—the great stabilizer. Never underestimate the training power of standing exercises, which can actually be more intense because the abs usually have to work harder to maintain balance through a broader range of motion and activity. In all standing exercises, maintain perfect posture, with your knees slightly bent. Sit into your leg base and feel your core as you move. Always begin slowly and speed up only as you master each move.

# STANDING TWIST (LEVEL 1)

Stand with your feet shoulder-width apart. Hold a medicine ball between your hands. Rotate, turning slowly to the left and then to the right. Start out with the ball close to your body. As you become familiar with the movement, extend the ball outward while holding your belly firm. Do not "suck in," but keep your torso elongated and abs firm.

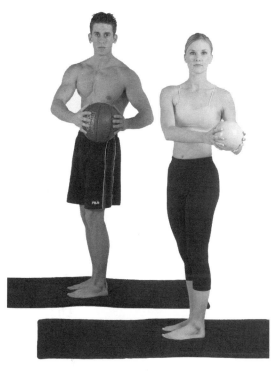

# CHOP WOOD (LEVEL 2)

Chop imaginary wood. Hold onto a medicine ball with both hands. Raise the ball above your head, turning to your right. Bring it down diagonally, close to your left hip. Alternate sides, from left to right.

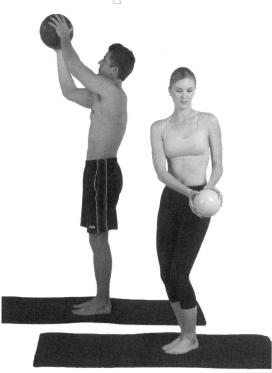

# OVERHEAD TOSS WITH PARTNER (LEVEL 3)

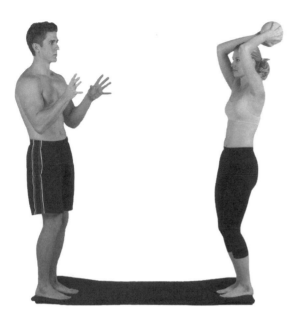

Lift a medicine ball overhead and bend back slightly to pull in the abdominal muscles. Then toss the ball to a partner. Make sure your partner is able and ready for your toss! The partner catches the ball and throws it back, forcing you to reach up. The movement strengthens your arms and torso.

# TRUNK LATERAL TOSS (LEVEL 3)

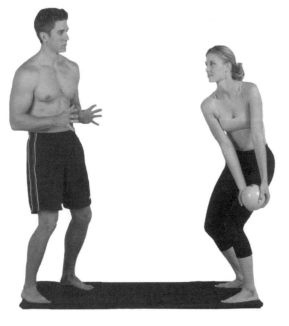

Stand facing a partner, then squat, leaning forward at a slight angle. Pull your abdomen tight and toss the ball underhand diagonally. You want to maintain a smooth motion during each throw. Your partner squats down and catches it low.

Stand and hold a medicine ball in both hands at arms' length overhead. Keep a slight bend in the elbows. Rotate your upper body from the waist as if you were drawing a large circle above you with the medicine ball. Do one set of 10 repetitions clockwise and one set counterclockwise. The emphasis is on the coordinated function of the entire torso musculature.

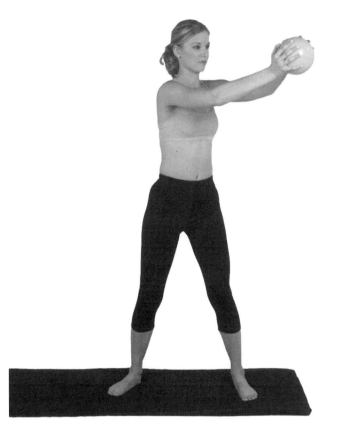

## SEATED OR SIT-UP EXERCISES

On all seated exercises, maintain perfect posture, focusing on your centered core and the movement surrounding it. Always start by performing each exercise slowly. Move faster as you master each movement. Never sacrifice form for speed.

## PARTNER SIT-UP (LEVEL 1)

Assume a bent-knee sit-up position and have a training partner stand on your feet to hold them down. Begin with your back off the floor. Your partner lightly tosses a medicine ball to you so that you catch it at chest level. Allow the force from the impact to push you almost to the floor. Just before your back touches, sit up forcefully and toss the ball back to your partner with a two-handed press.

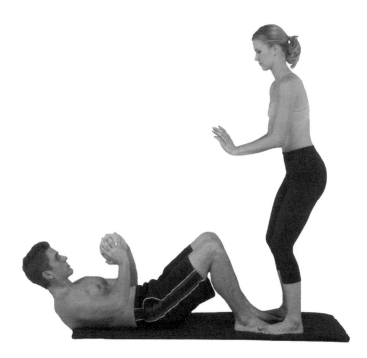

Assume a bent-knee sit-up position and have a training partner stand on your feet to hold them down. Begin with your back off the floor. Hold both arms outstretched over your head. Have your partner pass the ball lightly into your hands. Keeping your arms over your head, let the weight of the ball pull you back until your back almost touches the floor. Then sit up forcefully and pass the ball back to your partner.

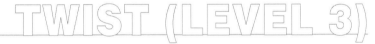

# TWIST (LEVEL 3)

Assume a sit-up position with your feet locked under a stationary object or with a partner holding them down. Sit back at a 45-degree angle to the floor. Hold a medicine ball in both hands straight out from your face. Keep your arms bent slightly. Twist your torso from side to side rhythmically. Concentrate on twisting to one side, suddenly reversing the momentum, and twisting to the other side. The emphasis is on the obliques and on isometric shoulder and lower-back strength.

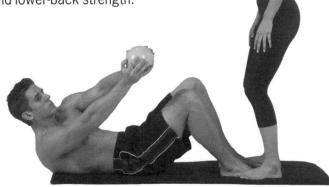

## Increasing Muscle Size

It takes more than 16 workouts to produce significant muscle fiber hypertrophy in your abdominal area. The size and strength of connective tissue, including ligaments and tendons, also increases, as does the sarcoplasm (muscle cell fluid).

Muscle takes up less space in your abdomen than fat. Fat bulges 18 percent more than an equal weight of muscle. Fat occupies 1.2 quarts (1.1 liters) per pound (0.5 kilogram), while muscle takes up just 1.0 quart (0.9 liters) per pound. Core training offsets any gains in muscle circumference by reducing fat, that is, as long as you do not increase your fat stores by wolfing down extra calories.

# MEDICINE-BALL PLYOMETRIC POWER TRAINING

Medicine-ball plyometrics help you train your entire body. You can mimic the sport-specific movements of your choice, such as throwing, catching, and so on. Unlike bench presses, medicine-ball drills work a variety of muscle groups at different angles as your body works to stabilize in space under varying conditions.

## MEDICINE-BALL CROSS AND THROW (LEVEL 1)

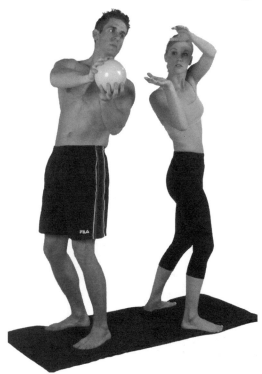

You can do this exercise standing or sitting. Hold the medicine ball in both hands with your arms extended. Bring the ball diagonally across to the right side of your body. Then quickly reverse directions and throw the ball over your left shoulder to your partner. Repeat on your other side.

# MEDICINE-BALL KICK-UP (LEVEL 2)

Stand with the medicine ball on the floor between your feet. Your ankles are "holding" the ball. Flex both knees and hips to "throw" the ball into your hands.

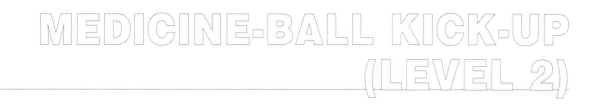

# MEDICINE-BALL PLYOMETRIC PUSH-UP (LEVEL 3)

Begin in a push-up position with both hands on the medicine ball. Push your arms off the ball and fall into a push-up position with the ball under your chest. Just as your hands hit the floor, hop back up to the start position. Keep your back flat throughout the exercise.

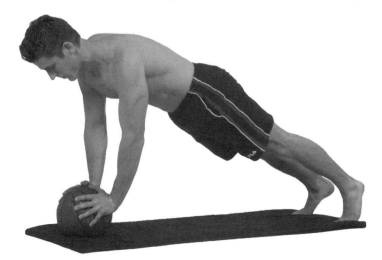

# DOUBLE BALL EXERCISES

Medicine balls combined with stability balls add two components to your training: power and stability. Be sure you are comfortable on a stability ball before you attempt the power drills. Begin slowly and progress gradually to ensure your safety. Get comfortable with the weight and texture of the medicine ball you are using as well. Gently toss and catch the ball yourself before you work on passing it with a partner. Allow your partner to do the same.

## MEDICINE-BALL PASS

While seated on a stability ball, have a partner chest-pass the medicine ball to you. As you catch the ball, you must stabilize yourself so that you do not fall off. Torso twists and overhead passes can also be done while you sit on the ball.

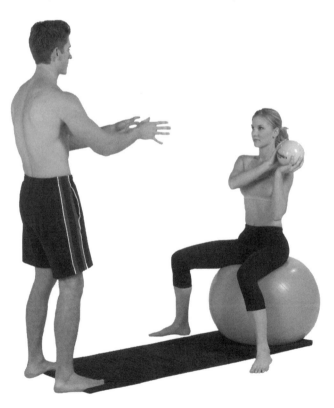

Sit on a stability ball with your feet anchored under a stationary object. Throw a medicine ball back and forth with a partner while performing sit-ups. This is a great way to develop strength for tennis, basketball, volleyball, baseball, or any sport that requires trunk flexion and extension.

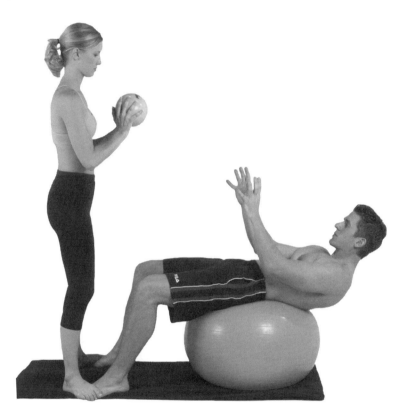

# ADVANCED BALANCE DRILL

Let's move on from the medicine ball to an intense leg and core drill that uses gravity and your own body's resistance. A great martial artist's forte when competing can be a high knee lift. The knee lift, especially sideways, is possible only with strength in the obliques, which can be enhanced by shadow boxing.

Begin by facing a full-length mirror. Stand in sparring position. Do one slow, low, front kick with each leg, and alternate with slow, low, round-house kicks (see chapter 9). Finally add slow, low, side kicks with each leg. Mix in easy punches with your kicks, as if you were shadow sparring. This aids your balance and strength progression.

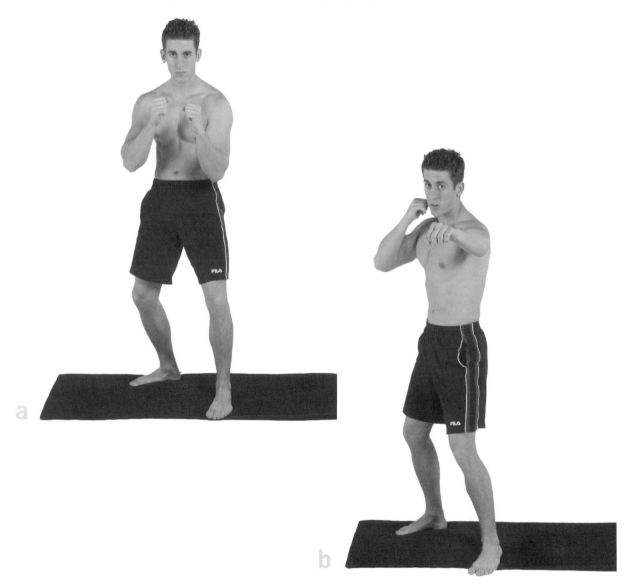

Shadow boxing helps develop the obliques. Begin in a good sparring position (a). Move through front, side, and back kicks, including some punches with the kicks (b).

# POWER PLYOMETRICS

Plyometric training takes advantage of the stretch–recoil effect in your muscles. When you stretch your muscles a little bit beyond resting length, like stretching a rubber band, stored energy causes a myotatic response. This allows you to explode through a movement faster and more powerfully than normal.

Your upper body and lower body are connected by your torso. Every time you jump, extend, or use your arms to propel you up into the air, your torso is the link in the power chain. Stability, jump, and plyometric training completely activates your abs, even though the exercises may not seem like ab exercises.

Plyometric training is an excellent method for improving your power. You can use plyometrics to train at a larger percentage of your aerobic capacity, so your workouts will eventually feel easier. These exercises can be performed individually or in a circuit:

1. Skip up a hill with an exaggerated knee lift and longer-than-usual stride. Jog down. Repeat 10 times.

2. Sprint up a hill, raising your knees high, and jog down. Repeat 10 times.

3. Stand on the grass with your feet shoulder-width apart. Crouch from your knees and hips, allowing your arms to swing backward close to your body for maximum energy. Explode from your leg base, allowing your arms to swing forward naturally, and bound as far as you can, landing resiliently. Perform 10 consecutive standing broad jumps.

4. Perform 10 consecutive very short hops across the grass.

5. Jump up and down 10 times as quickly as you can, keeping your feet as close to the ground as possible.

# 11

# ADVANCED ABS:
## Alternative Training

Hopefully, we have convinced you by now that activating your core is more than just tightening your abs. If we haven't made that clear to you, please go back and read everything again. Many of us desire some alternative training, which these workouts provide. These workouts can be your full-time everyday training if you prefer them.

## POOL WORKOUT

Certain moves can be done quite effectively in the pool. With the buoyancy and protection of the water, many people who feel unstable on land can excel in the water.

Water workouts are not limited only to those who feel unstable on land. These workouts can be as intense and advanced as land core conditioning but are wonderful for seniors, the physically challenged, or anyone who wants to vary the program.

Move to the water level specified in the exercise. In order to get an accurate photo, we had to shoot the exercise being done further out of the water than it should be done.

Stand in the water, opening your legs beyond shoulder-width, toes turned out 45 degrees. Lunge down into your leg base, keeping perfect lunge form (knees should not extend beyond your toes) (a). Your chest should now be at water level, arms resting on water surface, palms down. Keep at this level throughout the rest of the exercise. Now lunge to the left, without rising up out of the water, allowing your arms to flow and float naturally behind the rest of your body (b). Feel the natural resistance created by the water and the recoil and stretch as you flow from lunge to lunge. Your core is resiliently stabilizing and moving through different angles of movement. Try moving slowly for a few minutes, and then pick up the pace a little without assisting the movement with your arms. For a little more resistance to further challenge your core, let your hands turn sideways, forming little rudders.

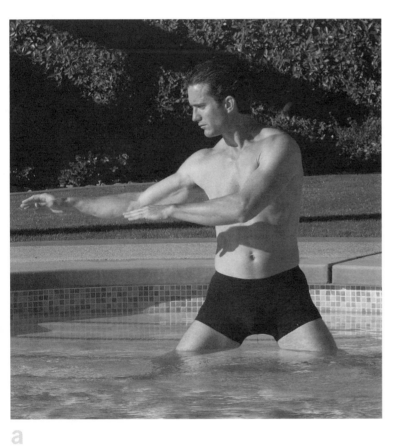

a

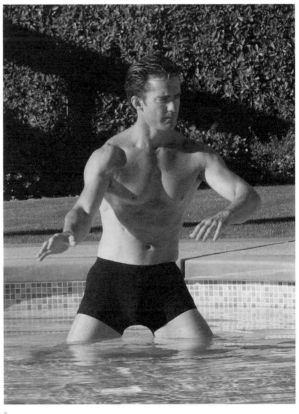

b

With your back to the pool wall (head above water, please), drape both arms over the pool edge (a). You can rest the back of your neck against the pool edge if you desire. Keeping your arms and shoulders relaxed, perform a bicycle-like rotating kick underwater to keep your body lengthened out and your pelvis up toward the water surface with little bend in the hips (b). Your head, neck, and shoulders should stay buoyantly relaxed above water. Try at first to maintain this movement for 30 seconds or more if you can, and then increase the duration by 10 extra seconds each week. Do at least five cycles with little rest in between. This exercise is good for the core and the back. You can play with it once you feel stable by turning your torso and legs from one side to the other for a fuller core experience.

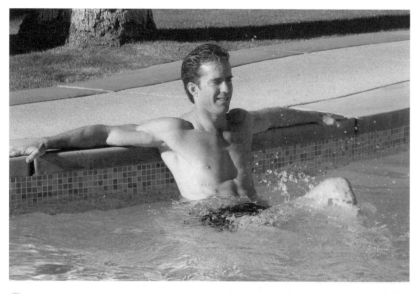

a

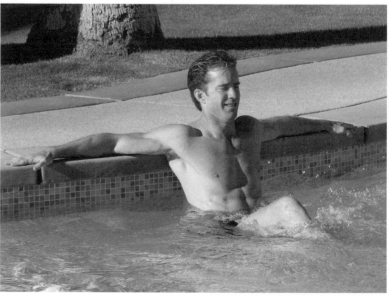

b

Standing in the water, lift one knee to the opposite elbow, feeling the resistance. To lengthen the range of motion, let your arm rest on top of the water, and extend the opposite leg sideways. Perform 10 repetitions in a row on one side before changing to the other side. Do three full cycles. For an advanced approach, try a plyometric jump in which the supporting leg leaves the pool floor as the other knee comes up toward the opposite elbow. Perform 10 reps on both sides.

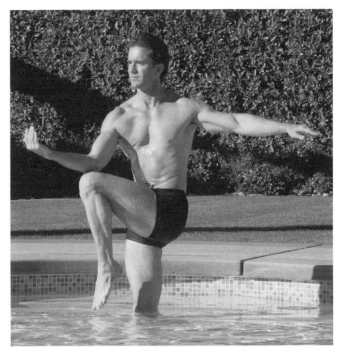

# DOUBLE-KNEE TUCK JUMP

Standing in the water at chest level, bend your knees and jump, extending your torso first, then bringing your knees up toward your chest. Let your arms naturally swing backward in the water to keep you upright. Try to land in the same place each time, working on coordination, balance, and core strength. Do two sets of 15 repetitions.

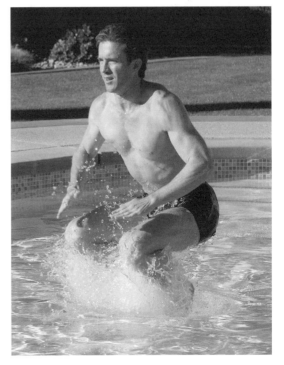

ADVANCED ABS: Alternative Training

With your knees bent up over the edge of the pool and your torso floating in the water, feel your core stability as your torso holds its own in the water. You will most likely begin by feeling this in the hip flexors; if so, try to relax and avoid grabbing with your legs. Instead let your arms float out, lifting your torso just slightly to feel the stability. Try to hold for 30 seconds to one minute, head always above water. This is an isometric exercise. Relax and lengthen to float, then slowly contract while breathing, and then slowly release. The range of motion is limited.

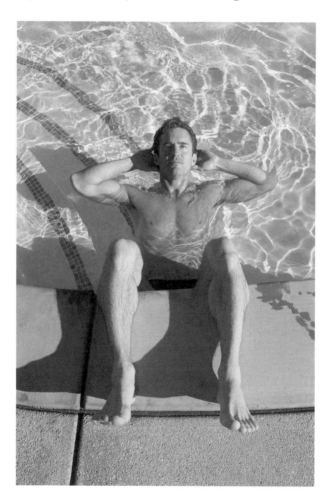

Drape your body over a hot tub wall (or something similar). Relax first, then slowly rise up into a back stability pose (a), hold for two seconds, then release. Try to achieve full-body balance, pointing your toes, using your arms less and less for stability as you feel more balanced in your back and buttocks with each repetition. Make sure to breathe as you go, performing 5 to 10 repetitions.

If you would rather not risk falling face-first into the pool or hot tub, turn around so your feet hang over the pool and you're lying face down at the side. Slowly rise into a back stability pose, spreading your arms and legs (b). Hold for two seconds and release. Perform 5 to 10 repetitions.

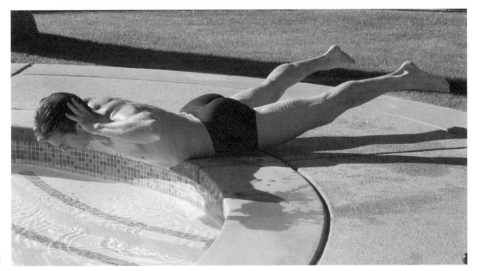

a

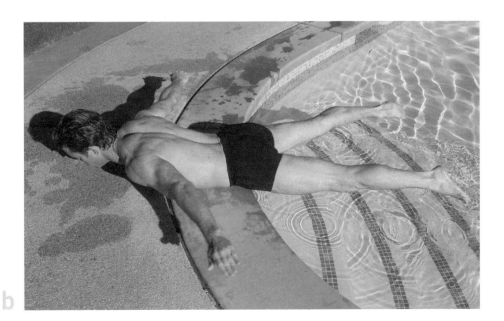

b

Sit with your buttocks on the edge of the first or second step of the pool, extending your legs out in front of you and leaning slightly back into a V position (a). Point your toes, bend your knees slightly, and alternate scissors kicks, crossing one ankle over the other and creating resistance in the water (b). Scissor-kick for 30 seconds, extend the legs up into a V position and hold for 5 seconds, breathe, and then continue the scissors kicks for 30 more seconds. To disengage the hip flexor a bit, turn the toes out slightly. The further back you can lean, the more you can target the core muscles. Do three cycles, and at the end hold a V-sit, breathe, lean to one side, hold, lean to the other side, hold, and relax.

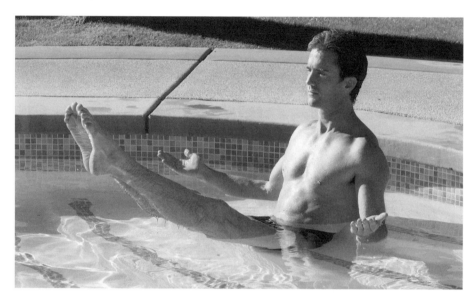

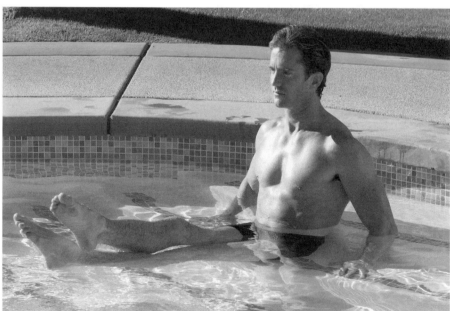

# STABILITY BALLS

Stability balls are also a different way to work your core. Like water core conditioning, they provide more all-around support to reduce risk of injury and increase comfort. The stability ball has been used as a physical therapy tool for years and is now also used quite effectively as a core conditioning tool.

When you perform movements on a stability ball, your abdominals, lower-back muscles, and other postural muscles are forced to contract to stabilize the body, while opposing muscle groups are allowed to lengthen in a fully supported position. This results in a much greater training effect. Move slowly through the following exercises, discovering your balance on this new apparatus. You can really feel the lengthening and the contraction of the core muscles. We recommend this kind of strength and stretch workout. Apply the same body awareness that you achieve on the stability ball to your everyday activities and workouts.

It is important to buy the right size ball and maintain the proper air pressure. The firmer the ball, the more difficult the exercise will be. If you are a beginner, overweight, older, or generally deconditioned, consider using a larger, softer ball. When you sit on the ball, your knees and hips should be at a 90-degree angle. Pick a color that you like. Believe it or not, color can be a motivating factor.

When exercising, let your ball fill the curve of your lower back, allowing your abdominal muscles to move through a greater range of motion to enhance both your strength and flexibility. You will discover that you must balance yourself so that you don't roll off the ball. Some of the following exercises can be done with a training partner. Try to balance on your own as much as possible. By doing so, you employ more muscles during your workout and also improve your overall balance.

In some exercises, you use muscles to anchor your body to the floor for stability. For example, during the supine inclined trunk curl, you can work the quads to a greater degree by bringing your buttocks closer to the floor. This places less resistance on the abdominals but requires the quads to stabilize the movement. The further away your seat is from the floor, the more work is required from your abdominals.

Drape your body over the ball (a). Keep your lower back on the middle of the ball. Your knees should be flexed 90 degrees, your thighs parallel to the floor. Execute normal crunches from this position (b). The ball allows a greater range of motion. These are excellent for torso strength, endurance, and stability.

During crunches, you can modify your arm position to adjust the resistance. The least resistance occurs when the arms are straight and outstretched along the sides of the body during the movement. A more difficult variation is to cross the arms against the chest. The most difficult variation is to touch the head with the fingers at a point just behind the ears. Avoid interlacing the fingers and clasping the hands behind the head, which can strain the cervical vertebrae and encourage participation from other muscles. Additional resistance (in the form of a medicine ball or weight plate) can be used when your body weight is no longer sufficient to cause an improvement in strength. If you use additional resistance, anchor the feet under an immovable object to stabilize your position.

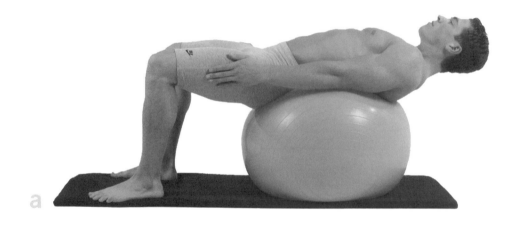

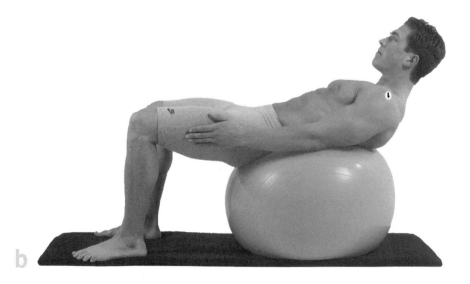

Lie on the ball, keeping your lower back on the middle of the ball (a). Your knees should be flexed 90 degrees, your thighs parallel to the floor. Slowly bring your ribcage toward your pubis (b). When you feel your abdominals contract, move slowly back to your original position. Perform 10 repetitions with perfect form. Add two repetitions a week as long as you can maintain perfect form for each repetition.

To increase intensity to level 2, add 10 repetitions. Add 10 more repetitions to increase to level 3.

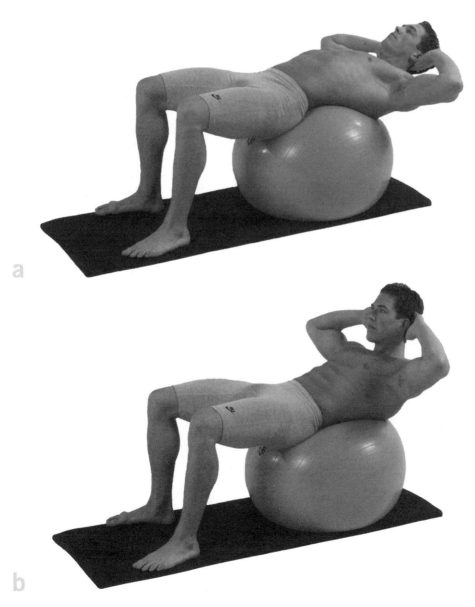

a

b

When you can perform 10 repetitions of level 1 exercises with perfect form, move on to level 2. When you can perform 10 repetitions at level 2 with perfect form, move on to level 3.

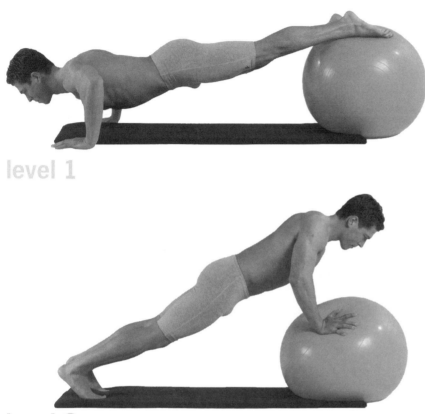

level 1

**Level 1:** Place the tops of your feet on the ball and your hands on the floor. Slowly lower your body to the floor, leading with your chest. Continue until your elbows are bent 90 degrees. Keep your back straight when performing push-ups; make sure that you don't arch or sag. Push yourself back into your original position. Perform 10 repetitions with perfect form.

level 2

**Level 2:** Assume a push-up position with the balls of your feet on the floor and your hands on the stability ball. Slowly lower your chest toward the ball until your elbows are bent at a 90-degree angle. Maintain perfect posture. Breathe, balance, and maintain your core strength. Push yourself back into your original position. Perform 10 repetitions with perfect form.

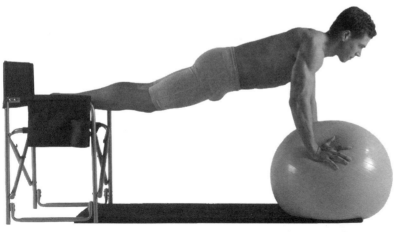

level 3

**Level 3:** Place your feet on a chair that is about the same height as the ball. Place your hands on the ball. Slowly lower your chest toward the ball until your elbows reach a 90-degree angle. Push yourself back up into your original position. Perform 10 repetitions with perfect form. Add two repetitions a week as long as you can maintain perfect form for each repetition. Start slowly and progress gradually, as this is very difficult.

Balance and stability can be highly developed using a stability ball. Its round shape provides an unstable base from which to perform various exercises. As a result, stabilizer muscles strengthen, and kinesthetic awareness improves.

**Level 1:** Kneel on the stability ball with both knees, and hold the position for intervals of 30 seconds to one minute. Have a training partner spot you in case you fall. When this becomes easy, try to hold the position with your eyes closed.

**Level 2:** Hold the ball straight out from your chest with both hands. Keep your elbows soft. Step forward into a deep lunge, and twist your torso to the side of the forward leg. Twist back as you step back into the starting position. Repeat on the other side. This exercise develops total-body balance.

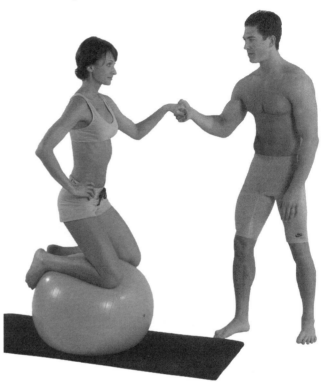

level 1

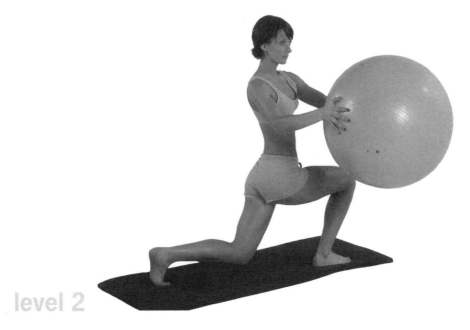

level 2

Position yourself on the ball as you would when performing crunches. Grasp a medicine ball with both hands. Keeping your elbows extended and arms perpendicular to your torso, rotate to either side. Maintain neutral head and neck position. Also, do not allow your pelvis to rotate with your torso as you twist from side to side, as this unloads the oblique muscles. You can increase the difficulty of the exercise by using a heavier medicine ball, increasing the speed of the movement, or positioning yourself farther back on the ball (you may need to anchor your feet to prevent falling backward over the ball).

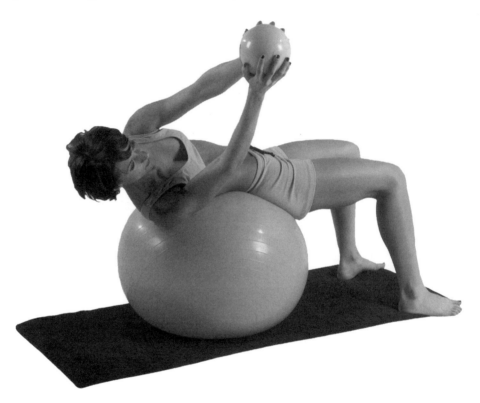

From a kneeling position with a ball directly in front of you, place your clasped hands on top of the ball (a). Extend yourself forward until your hips, shoulders, and elbows are fully extended (b). Return to the starting position by reversing the motion. As you extend, the increased load on your abs causes the curve of your low back to tend to increase. The goal is to counteract this tendency by tucking your pelvis under as you extend. If you are unable to maintain constant low-back curvature during this exercise, you'll need to spend more time working on the pelvic tilt described in chapter 6.

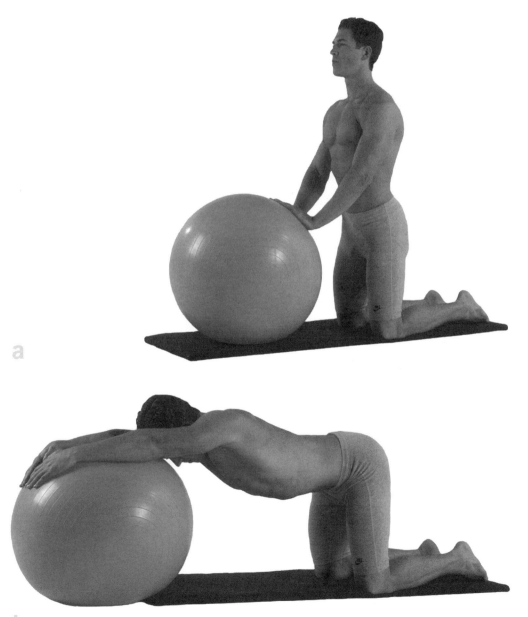

a

b

# glossary

**abdominal fat**—Nobody wants it, but men particularly tend to store fat in the abdomen (especially if beer and potato chips are involved). Fortunately, exercise releases epinephrine, which reacts with hormone-sensitive lipase to help reduce fat around the waist.

**abdominals (or abs)**—Everybody wants to see their abdominals, the flat, bandlike muscles on the front of the trunk. These muscles connect the pelvis to the rib cage. They consist of the rectus abdominis, external and internal obliques, and transversus abdominis.

**abductors**—The outer-thigh muscles, including the tensor fasciae latae and gluteus medius.

**actin**—No, we do not mean actin' school. Actin is one of the fibrous protein components of muscle tissue that, with myosin, forms a crossbridge to contract muscle.

**active isolated (AI) stretching**—A type of stretching in which the antagonist (or opposing) muscle is contracted for two seconds prior to stretching the agonist muscle for two seconds. As many as 10 repetitions of each stretch can be done. The purpose of AI stretching is to inhibit the stretch reflex.

**active recovery**—If you really want to hurt, run a sprint, and then sit instead of actively recovering. Toxins accumulate in muscles after exercise. These metabolites (waste products) are drastically reduced if you perform some type of activity after your workout. Walking, pedaling, or light jogging for 10 to 15 minutes greatly increases the breakdown of metabolites to reduce unwanted stiffness and soreness.

**adaptation**—Improvement; the adjustment of the body or mind to achieve greater fitness. Conditioning usually occurs as a result of more intense training. You have to work hard so your body will adapt to the extra stress and you can move to the next level of training.

**adductors**—The inner-thigh muscles, including the adductor magnus, adductor longus, adductor brevis, and gracilis.

**adenosine triphosphate (ATP)**—An organic molecule used as a storage form of energy in cells. It is the final phase in the transfer of food energy to work performed by muscle. ATP must be present in muscle cells for a contraction to occur.

**aerobic activities**—*Aerobic* means "with oxygen." Aerobic activities include walking, running, jogging, cycling, and swimming, which use large muscle groups at moderate intensities to allow the body to use oxygen to supply energy and maintain a steady state of exercise for more than a few minutes.

**agonist**—This is not about agony unless you hate weight training. An agonist is a muscle that directly engages in an action around a joint. The antagonist provides the opposite action.

**anaerobic exercise**—Usually short-term, high-intensity exercise. *Anaerobic* means "without oxygen." The fuels for this quick exercise are ATP, creatine phosphate, and glycogen. Weightlifting, sprinting, basketball, racquetball, and tennis are anaerobic activities.

**antagonist**—Your spouse. No, really it's a muscle that provides an opposing action to the action of another muscle (the agonist) around a joint. For example, the antagonist of the biceps is the triceps.

**biceps**—The muscles on the front of the upper arm (think of Popeye), including the biceps brachii, brachialis, and brachioradialis.

**body fat**—The fat in the body. The lower your percentage of body fat, the more muscular you appear. Percentage body fat is the ratio of fat to lean body mass (that is, muscle, bone, and so on). Men can achieve as little as 3 percent fat, and women, 12 percent, but these are extremes. A reasonable goal for men is 10 to 15 percent fat; for women, 15 to 20 percent.

**bodybuilding**—The application of weight training and nutrition to enhance musculature and physical appearance. A person can be a bodybuilder without being a huge hulk.

**calorie**—Scientifically speaking, a calorie is the amount of energy required to raise the temperature of one gram of water one degree Celsius. Calories don't have to be your enemy. All of your bodily functions require calories.

**carbohydrate**—Carbohydrates are not to be avoided, as some of the latest fad diets would have you believe. A carbohydrate contains carbon, hydrogen, and oxygen. It is an efficient source of energy for your cells. It yields 4.1 calories per gram. Sources of carbohydrates include potatoes, rice, beans, peas, corn, fruits, and grains. Processed carbohydrates are calorically denser; for the same quantity of food they have a lot more calories. Processed carbohydrates include pasta, bagels, and cereals. Carbs supply your muscles with energy to complete your workout.

**cardio versus strength training**—Which should you do first? If you're doing both, who cares which one goes first? But if you do care, do your strength training first. This way, you can recycle that lactic acid from your weight work for energy during your cardio workout.

**conditioning**—A general fitness term that refers to improving your health through physical training.

**contraction**—You can have a contraction whether you're male or female. The shortening of a muscle caused by the crossbridging and coming together of actin and myosin filaments.

**cool-down**—The gradual reduction in the intensity of exercise. The purpose of the cool-down is to prevent soreness and to allow the heart rate, hormones, blood pressure, and all physiological processes to return to their pre-exercise condition. A cool-down also helps prevent blood pooling in the legs and may reduce muscular soreness.

**cramp**—You've probably had one of these when you're trying to fall asleep. All of a sudden, without warning, your calf muscle knots up into a painful spasm. This is a cramp. Sometimes it's your body's way of preventing you from participating in an activity for which your muscles aren't ready. Other times it's a signal that you have an electrolyte imbalance.

**creatine phosphate (CP)**—A form of creatine, the magic muscle builder; an organic compound found in your muscle fibers that breaks down to produce ATP to energize your workout and life.

**crossbridges**—Don't burn your crossbridges. They contract the muscle fibers and are created by actin and myosin filaments' "grabbing" each other and pulling together.

**cross-training**—In cross-training, two or more types of exercise are performed in a single workout or used alternately in successive workouts. For example, a distance cyclist may run twice a week, stretch daily, and lift weights occasionally.

**crunch**—A tilt-curl-uncurl-untilt flexion and extension of your spine from a supine (on your back) position. This overrated exercise isolates your abdominals and prevents your hip flexors (iliopsoas) from contracting. You won't lose fat doing crunches.

**deltoids**—The large triangular shoulder muscles that include the anterior deltoid, medial deltoid, and posterior deltoid. They raise (abduct) the arm away from the body to the side.

**detraining**—Losing the benefits of your training by not exercising. Use it or lose it.

**dumbbell**—Not that obnoxious upstairs neighbor. Hand weights generally used by professional bodybuilders as their preferred resistance devices.

**eating after exercise**—A way to feel better after a workout. The carbohydrate window of opportunity is a 15-minute period after a workout when the muscles are most receptive to recovering nutrients. Simple carbohydrates will do. Exercise provides a greater of volume of blood to the muscles. The blood carries carbohydrates that are absorbed from the stomach. This causes maximum nutrient reabsorption into your muscles, providing a more rapid recovery from exercise.

**electrolytes**—Sodium, potassium, chloride, calcium, magnesium, and other minerals that provide conductivity to help fluid pass through cellular membranes.

**erector spinae**—A long muscle that extends up the back from the pelvis to the bony processes of the vertebrae, the rib cage, and upper parts of the spine.

**external obliques**—The visible (if a layer of fat is not covering them) "hands in the front pocket" abdominal muscles. These muscles help you pull and twist the torso or reach across your body as you lean forward.

**fast-twitch (type IIb) muscle fibers**—White, glycolytic muscle fibers that contract quickly and forcefully and are valuable for high-intensity, short-duration activities.

**fiber type**—Your parents are responsible for your fiber type. You will never be as fast as Donovan Bailey if you were not blessed with a preponderance of fast-twitch fibers. Your core is made up of a combination of fast-twitch and slow-twitch fibers, so it's beneficial to train both using the exercises in this book.

**flexibility**—The range of motion around a joint.

**free weights**—See also *dumbbell*. These weights are not free of charge. Free weights allow you to follow the natural line of pull of your muscles and require you to use stabilizer muscles to balance the weight. Free weights also let you prestretch your muscles to the optimal length (1.2 times their resting length) just before you do a lift. These are some of the reasons that professional bodybuilders seem to prefer free weights over machines.

**gastrocnemius (calf muscle)**—The long, sleek muscle on the back of the lower leg.

**gluteals (glutes)**—The buttocks; hip extensors that include the gluteus maximus, medius, and minimus.

**glycogen**—Sugar in muscle; the energy source that muscles prefer; a storage form of carbohydrate in liver and muscle. Don't run out of this or you'll feel lethargic and "bonk." Glycogen is converted to glucose to be used by muscles for energy.

**golgi tendon organ**—If you can override your golgi tendon organ, you can lift a car. When you stretch a muscle, you can activate your golgi tendon organ. Your golgi tendon organ relaxes the muscle so that it will not become injured. For example, if you are trying to lift a weight off of the floor and it is too heavy for your muscles to support, your golgi tendon organ will cause your muscles to relax and you will drop the weight.

**hamstrings**—The large muscles in the back of the upper leg.

**hypertrophy**—Usually used to refer to an increase in muscle size. An increase in a body part's or organ's (usually muscle's) size or in the amount of water, fat, satellite cells, or other substances in response to highly specific forms of stress.

**iliopsoas**—Hip flexor muscle located inside the pelvis on the side of the lumbar vertebrae and attached from the lumbar vertebrae to the thigh bone. It helps to lift the knee.

**internal obliques**—Abdominal muscles located beneath the external obliques and shaped like a rooftop. The right internal oblique turns the torso to the right, and the left turns the torso to the left.

**isometric**—Pushing against an immovable object. In an isometric contraction, the muscles contract without movement. An isometric contraction is a static contraction.

**lactate threshold**—Anaerobic threshold or OBLA (onset of blood lactate). This is where lactic acid cannot be eliminated as fast as it is being produced causing hydrogen ions to cause your muscles to burn while you are huffing and puffing.

**lactic acid**—Not the bad guy of exercise as once thought. Lactic acid is one of the by-products of muscle metabolism. It causes that burning sensation when you exercise hard. If you get too much lactate in your muscles, they decide to slow down and eventually quit working. It is a good idea to use active recovery during interval training so that all the accumulated lactate can be converted into glycogen to prepare you for your next bout of exercise.

**latissimus dorsi (lat)**—A long, wide muscle of the back. When it is developed, it takes the shape of wings.

**lower abs**—The part of the rectus abdominis below the belly button.

**motor unit**—A motor neuron and all of the muscle fibers it innervates. In your calf muscle, one neuron can activate as many as 1,000 fibers. But in your eye, where fine motor movement is required, one nerve cell may control only three fibers.

**muscle**—Muscle is precious. Seventy-five percent of your muscle is water, 20 percent is protein, and 5 percent minerals. You have more than 400 voluntary muscles in your body. Muscle makes up about half of your body weight. The more muscle you have, the more calories your body burns because muscle is metabolically active.

**muscle definition**—Visible muscularity with a minimum of subcutaneous body fat. Definition is not about high-repetition, low-weight workouts. Most people think the way to lose the fat between your skin and muscle is to lift light weights and perform lots of repetitions. But muscular definition is a function of your eating, aerobics, and full-body resistance-training program. You may do hundreds of repetitions of crunches, but if a layer of fat surrounds your abdominals (abs), you will never see your six-pack.

**myofibril**—The part of your muscle fiber that actually shortens when it contracts. It is composed of actin and myosin filaments.

**myosin**—A thick filament that crossbridges with the thin actin filaments to produce a muscular contraction.

**obliques**—Muscles on the sides of the abdomen that rotate and flex the trunk. See also *external obliques* and *internal obliques.*

**overload**—Subjecting a part of your body to loads greater than it is accustomed to. This improves performance as the body adapts to the increased intensity or duration.

**overtraining**—Don't forget to rest. The same motivation that you have to train hard and perform well can get you into trouble. Not allowing enough recovery between training sessions causes diminishing returns in your exercise program. Runners are notorious for overtraining. Day after day of pounding can adversely affect your joints, ligaments, and tendons. Overtraining can also lead to debilitating and often long-term fatigue that can severely limit your performance and fitness. One way to combat overtraining is to cross-train (see also cross-training).

**pectorals (pecs)**—Chest muscles, including the pectoralis major and pectoralis minor.

**periodization**—A fancy word for a well-thought-out exercise program. A training program segmented into weeks (microcycle), months (mesocycle), and years (macrocycle). Each training cycle helps you set short-term goals that ultimately help you reach your long-term goals.

**plyometrics**—Bounding drills. A stretch prior to a jump preloads your muscle, using the stretch reflex to create a myotatic response to recruit more muscle fibers for increased power in your jump.

**prone**—Lying face down.

**proprioception**—Balance.

**proprioceptive neuromuscular facilitation (PNF) stretch**—This one really works. A stretching technique designed to contract a muscle just prior to stretching it. The Golgi tendon organ senses the contraction and automatically relaxes that muscle, so you can stretch farther.

**proprioceptor**—Sense organs (including muscle spindles and Golgi tendon organs) found in your muscles, tendons, joints, and skin that help you to remain balanced within your environment.

**pursed-lipped breathing**—Slow exhalation by puckering your lips as if you were whistling. Martial artists and pregnant women use this type of breathing.

**quadriceps (quads)**—A group of four thigh muscles: rectus femoris, vastus lateralis, vastus medialis, and vastus intermedius. This muscle group extends the knee.

**rectus abdominis (six-pack)**—A long, straplike muscle extending from the lower and middle ribcage to the pubis. It lifts you from a lying to a sitting position.

**rhomboids**—Muscles between the shoulder blades. They help keep the shoulders back.

**ripped**—Showing good muscle definition.

**set**—A group of consecutive repetitions.

**slow-twitch (type I) muscle fibers**—Red, oxidative muscle fibers that contract slowly for endurance-type activities. They are not very powerful, but they can contract for long periods.

**soleus**—The muscle underneath your calf muscle. It adds volume to your lower leg. It is made up of predominantly slow-twitch muscle fibers.

**speed work**—Ready to rumble? Try speed work, a series of short, fast intervals designed to improve speed.

**spot reduction**—A common fitness myth that you can lose fat in one area of your body by performing targeted exercises specific to that area (for example, that ab exercises alone can reduce a spare tire around the waist). Through exercise, you lose fat over your entire body, not just in one place.

**static stretching**—Holding a stretch at a point of tension.

**stress**—Not always a bad thing. Stress is the body's response to any demand. Just staying alive puts demands on your body, so you are always under stress. This type of stress cannot be avoided. Even while you sleep, your body continues to function. Unhealthy stress caused by anxiety is linked to problems like high blood pressure and heart disease. It also exacerbates headaches, backaches, and digestive troubles. Stress can make your body aches more painful, your stomach queasy, or worsen any symptoms, no matter what the original cause. Unhealthy stress can also make a person downright unpleasant. But there is good stress, too. Think of the good feeling you have when you reach the next level in your exercise program. You are able to reach the next level because your body has adapted to the stress you put on it.

**stretching**—Feels so good afterwards. Stretching is optimally lengthening a muscle to increase the flexibility of that musculotendinous unit. A combination of massage and stretching is the perfect medicine for tightened muscles after a workout. Use massage to relax your muscles. Now your muscle is prepared for recovery stretching. This keeps your muscles from tightening and shortens recovery time.

**stretch reflex**—Like a rubber band effect. When muscle spindles sense a stretch, they cause a reflexive contraction of that muscle so the stretch won't cause damage. When you stretch a muscle too hard or too fast, it will contract to protect itself.

**supine**—Lying on your back.

**taper down**—Cool down.

**training**—Stressing the body to increase the ability to do a task.

**training effect**—You have to work to get results. When you train to overload your body, your body adapts by getting stronger. The training effect is the adaption to the overload.

**training motivation**—Get a healthy perspective. Make friends with your body. It deserves your kindness. Then make better choices. Walk away from sedentary life. Include more physical activity and healthier foods in your day. Soon you'll feel better both mentally and physically.

**transversus abdominis**—If you need to upchuck, you need your transversus abdominis. The transversus abdominis is an abdominal muscle that lies beneath the obliques. It contracts forcefully when you cough, sneeze, vomit, or defecate.

**trapezius (trap, gorilla muscle)**—The muscle of the upper shoulder and the side of the neck.

**triceps brachii (triceps, horseshoe muscle)**—The muscle in the back of your arm that extends your elbow.

**upper abs**—Rectus abdominis muscles above the belly button.

**vitamin**—Vitamins don't increase energy. They assist chemical reactions in your body. There are 13 known vitamins. Four are fat-soluble—A, D, E, and K; your body is able to store these in amounts large enough to last for months. There are nine water-soluble vitamins—C (ascorbic acid) and the B-complex vitamins: $B_1$ (thiamin), $B_2$ (riboflavin), $B_6$ (pyridoxine), $B_{12}$, niacin, folic acid, biotin, and pantothenic acid. Your body needs replenishment of these vitamins regularly.

**warm-up**—A gradual increase in the intensity of exercise that allows physiological processes to prepare for greater energy output. Don't forget your warm-up. A thorough warm-up increases body temperature, increases the elasticity and contractility of the muscles, and increases synovial fluid in the joints by 5 to 10 percent. Warm up before training. Stretch after your workout, when your muscles are thoroughly heated up.

# bibliography

Bogduk, N. 1999. *Clinical anatomy of the lumbar spine and sacrum* (3rd ed.). New York: Churchill Livingstone.

Bogduk, N., and Towmey, L.T. 1991. *Clinical anatomy of the lumbar spine* (2nd ed.). New York: Churchill Livingstone.

Chek, P. The outer unit. Available: **www.ptonthenet.com**.

Cholewicki, J., Juluru, K., and McGill, S. 1999. Intra-abdominal pressure mechanism for stabilizing the lumbar spine. *Journal of Biomechanics* 32:13-17.

Cole, S. 2000. *Tai chi training: Instructor training manual.* Palm Springs, Calif., and New Hope, Pa.: Millennium Fitness and AAAI/ISMA.

Fleck, S., and Kraemer, W. 1987. *Designing resistance training programs.* Champaign, IL: Human Kinetics.

Hodges, P.W., and Richardson, C.A. 1997. Contraction of the abdominal muscles associated with movement of the lower limb. *Physical Therapy* 77(2):132-142.

Howley, E., and Franks, B.D. 1992. *Health and fitness instructor's handbook* (2nd ed.). Champaign, IL: Human Kinetics.

Lee, D. 1999. *The pelvic girdle: An approach to the examination and treatment of the lumbo-pelvic-hip region* (2nd ed.). New York: Churchill Livingstone.

National Strength and Conditioning Association. 1994. *Essentials of strength and conditioning.* Edited by T. Baechle. Champaign, IL: Human Kinetics.

Richardson, C.A., and Jull, G.A. 1995. Muscle control—pain control. What exercises would you prescribe? *Manual Therapy* 1:2-10.

# about the authors

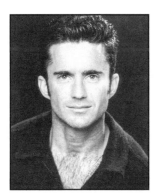

**Scott Cole** burst onto the fitness scene as a National Aerobic Champion and star of the best-selling videos *Abs of Steel, Best Abs on Earth, Millennium Stretch,* and now the *Discover Tai Chi* series. Combining brains and brawn, Scott has lifted spirits in over 30 countries as a lecturer/speaker. He has been featured in over 300 magazines, Web sites, and TV shows, including "Live with Regis and Kelly," "HARD COPY," "Good Day NY," *WebMD, USA Today, LA Times, SHAPE, GQ, Men's Fitness,* and more. His Hollywood clients include Christian Bale (*American Psycho*) and Gena Lee Nolin (*Baywatch*). Cole's professional accomplishments include being named one of IDEA's Top Five Fitness Instructors in the world, being an AFAA Notable (for his work with abused children and HIV/AIDS patients), and presenting at the Olympic Center in Moscow. He currently resides in Palm Springs, California, and can be contacted at **www.scottcole.com**.

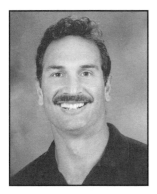

**Tom Seabourne**, PhD, has over 30 years of experience in the fitness industry. He has been featured on many television shows and in magazine articles, including *Sports Illustrated* as Athlete of the Month, *Men's Fitness* as Sportsman of the Month, and *Men's Exercise* as Mr. Fitness. Cycling and martial arts are among his chief interests. He holds several distance records in ultra cycling as well as a third-dan black belt in karate and taekwondo. He is also a two-time AAU national taekwondo champion.

Certified by the American Council on Exercise and the American College of Sports Medicine, Seabourne has written 10 previous books and more than 200 magazine articles. He resides in Mt. Pleasant, Texas, and teaches at Texas A&M University and Northeast Texas Community College.